NATURAL MEDICINE FOR HORSES

Home Remedies and Natural Healing

Horse Riding and Management Series

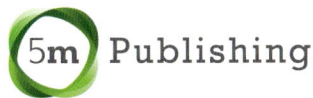
5m Publishing

Published by
5M Publishing Ltd,
Benchmark House,
8 Smithy Wood Drive,
Sheffield, S35 1QN, UK
Tel: +44 (0) 1234 81 81 80
www.5mpublishing.com

A catalogue record for this book is available from the British Library

ISBN 978-1-910455-10-4

Book layout by
Keystroke, Station Road, Codsall, Wolverhampton

Printed by Replika Press Pvt. Ltd, India

Photos by Dietmar Aichele, Hans D. Dossenbach, Monika Dossenbach, Werner Ernst, John Foxx Images, Klaus-Jürgen Guni, Volker Greiner, Höller, Irene Hohe, Petra Hülck, Sabine Küpper, Hans Kuczka, Hans E. Laux, Lothar Lenz, Masterhorse, Bernhard Metzler, Manfred Pforr, Dagmar Picard, Peter Prohn, Reinhard-Tierfoto, Ralf Roppelt, Marc Rühl, Christof Salata, Bernd Schellhammer, Peter Schönfelder, Edgar Schöpal, Maximilian Schreiner, Christiane Slawik, Horst Streitfeld/Kosmos, Sabine Stuewer, Felix von Döring, Cornelia Wittek

NATURAL MEDICINE FOR HORSES

Home Remedies and Natural Healing

Horse Riding and Management Series

CORNELIA WITTEK

Translated by John Kinory

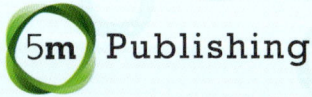

5m Publishing

Contents

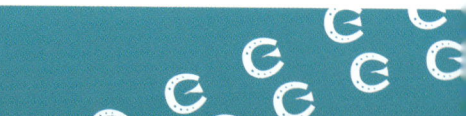

A varied diet   161

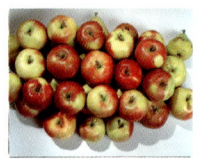

Year-round health   170

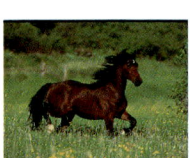

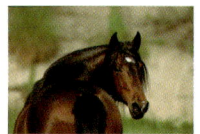

Dedication

I dedicate this book to all my horses, but especially to my two favourites Polly and Kaitra. For well over twenty years they shared my life, filled my leisure time with joy and happiness, helped me to relieve stress, helped us to raise our children and laid the foundation stone for this book. Thank you!

Further thanks go to my editor Alexandra Haungs, without whose capable assistance this book would never have happened.

Thank you to my family, in particular my daughter Steffi who came up with the idea for this book.

Many thanks to Dr. Thomas Sander, who offered me his help without prompting, to Selma Keienburg, Dagmar Picard and to the diligent computer experts Christa Löschmann and Elke Holstein. And very special thanks go to the best of all stable-hands, Werner Wetzel.

Heartfelt thanks too, go to my friends Judith and Klaus Balkenhol for the foreword.

Cornelia Wittek

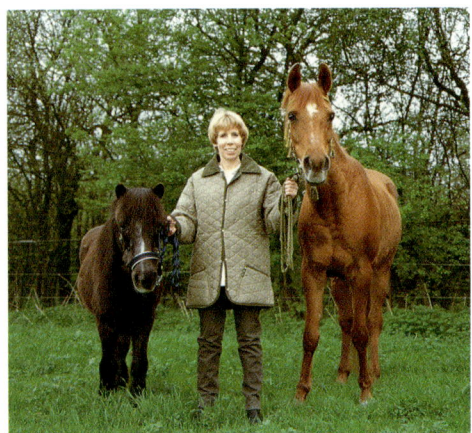

The publisher and translator wish to thank Deborah Graf, Jacqui Birnie, Alison Layland and Meryl Clarke for their help and advice with the translation of equine and medical terminology.

Foreword

Horses enhance our leisure time, enrich our lives, compete with us as partners in sporting events. We, as riders and horse keepers, bear responsibility for our animals. Healthy horses, full of joie de vivre, require appropriate husbandry, care and training.

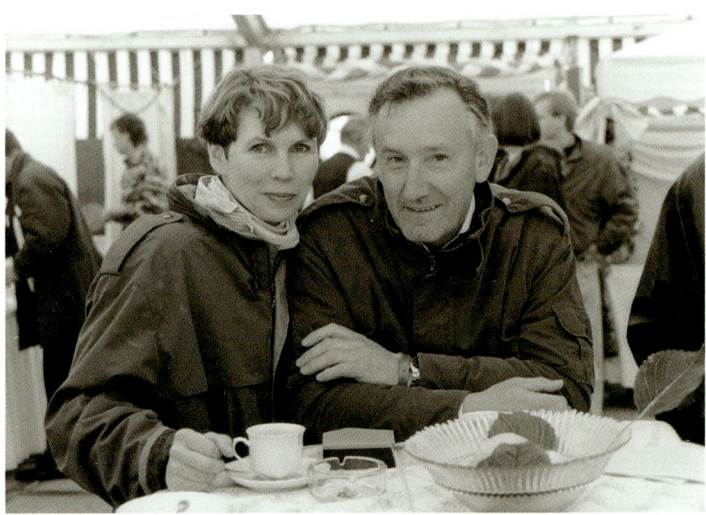

Every horse is an individual and wishes to be treated as such. In particular, our 'top athletes' are highly sensitive creatures who want to be looked after individually. Physical and mental well-being are an essential basis for the motivation of our horses. Our four-legged friends too are sometimes 'out of sorts', are plagued by minor ailments or suffer from stress and nervousness. Nobody notices this more quickly than the rider, owner or carer.

With proven home remedies and natural healing methods which have been helping us humans for a long time, you can also help your horse in such cases and contribute to its well-being. It goes without saying that vinegar, comfrey and ginseng are no substitute for the vet; but we always try in our stable, as far as possible, to use tried and tested home and natural remedies to improve the vitality of our horses, or to accompany the veterinary treatment and support it.

This book will tell you in detail how, and with the help of which natural remedies, you can care for your horse and treat it, and what the vet has to say about this.

Cornelia Wittek, the author of this book, is a long-time friend of our family and has already helped us and our horses a great deal with her knowledge and her experience in this field. We are delighted that she has now written down her expertise, thus making it accessible to a wider circle of horse lovers. She has managed to produce a book that is equally 'healthy' for horse and rider. We hope that you will derive much pleasure from reading and looking up information in it, and wish your horses health, success and a long and happy life.

Klaus and Judith Balkenhol

Headway charity disclaimer

The books in the 'Horse Riding and Management Series' were originally published in Germany. The photos used in the books are taken from the German books and in some cases show riders not wearing protective helmets. The law on wearing protective headgear differs between countries, states and equestrian disciplines. However, it is strongly advised that all riders wear a properly fitting, CE-approved helmet at all times when riding, whether on private or public ground, for all riding activities. The UK Highway Code makes it clear that children under the age of 14 must wear a helmet that complies with the Regulations, and other riders should also follow these requirements. This applies to roads, bridleways, footpaths, cycle paths and other roadways.

5m have partnered with Headway – the brain injury association on this issue to highlight the importance of children and adults wearing appropriate head protection while riding. The following statement has been provided by Headway:

> Headway, the UK-wide charity that supports people affected by brain injury, strongly advises riders of all ages and abilities to wear hats with straps that meet British standards.
>
> We all think 'it will never happen to me', but the reality is that an accident can happen to anyone at any time, with all riders at risk – regardless of age or experience.
>
> If worn correctly, riding hats are effective at preventing head and brain injuries, the effects of which can be devastating and last a lifetime.
>
> To all horse and pony riders, we simply say: Please, use your head, use a hat.

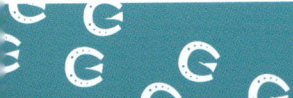

For further information about brain injury and how Headway helps those affected, or to make a donation to the charity, please visit www.headway.org.uk or call the freephone helpline on 0808 800 2244.

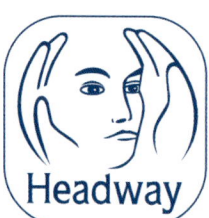

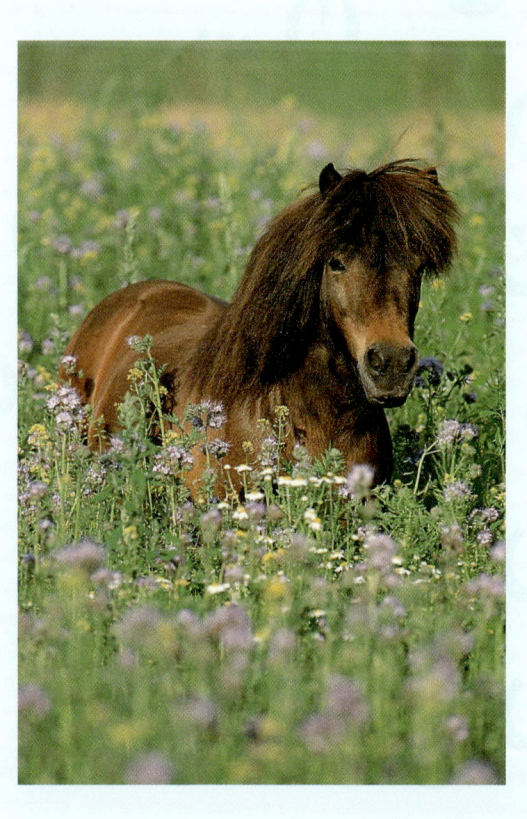

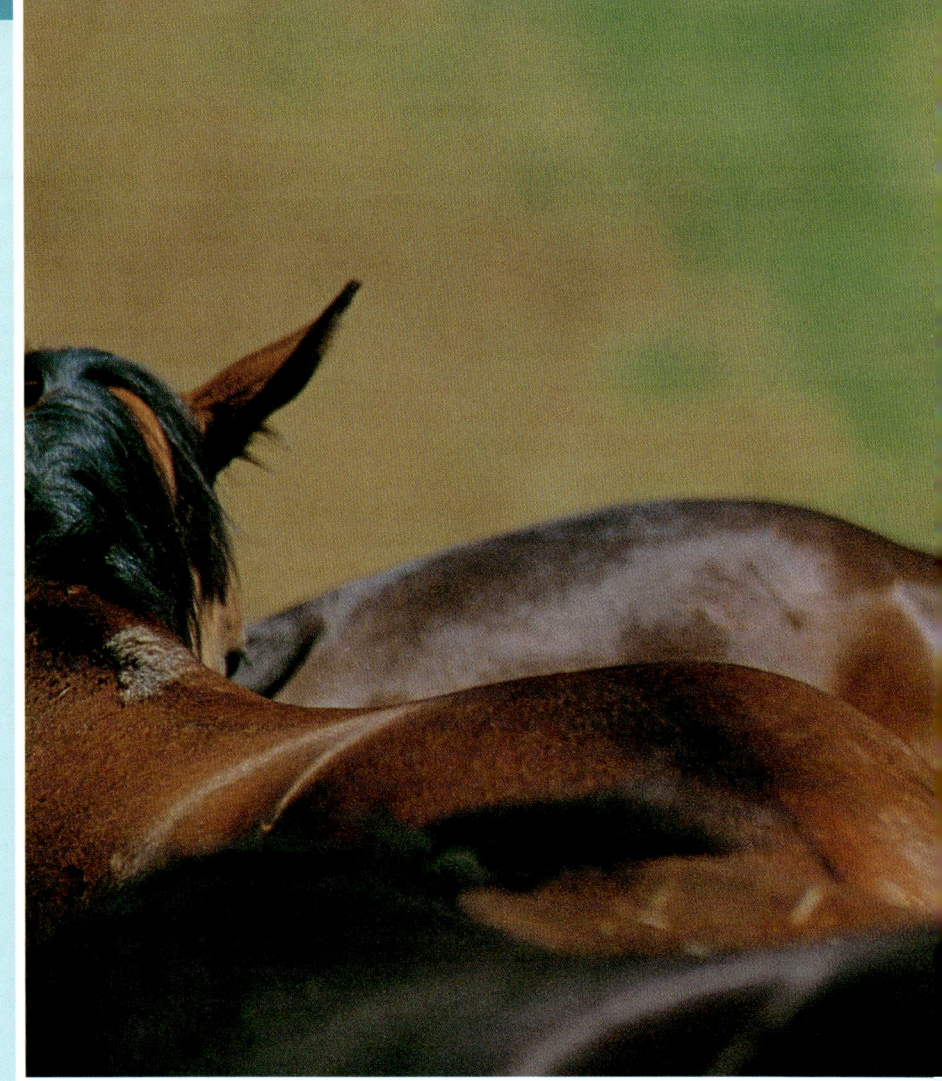

Gentle help
from nature

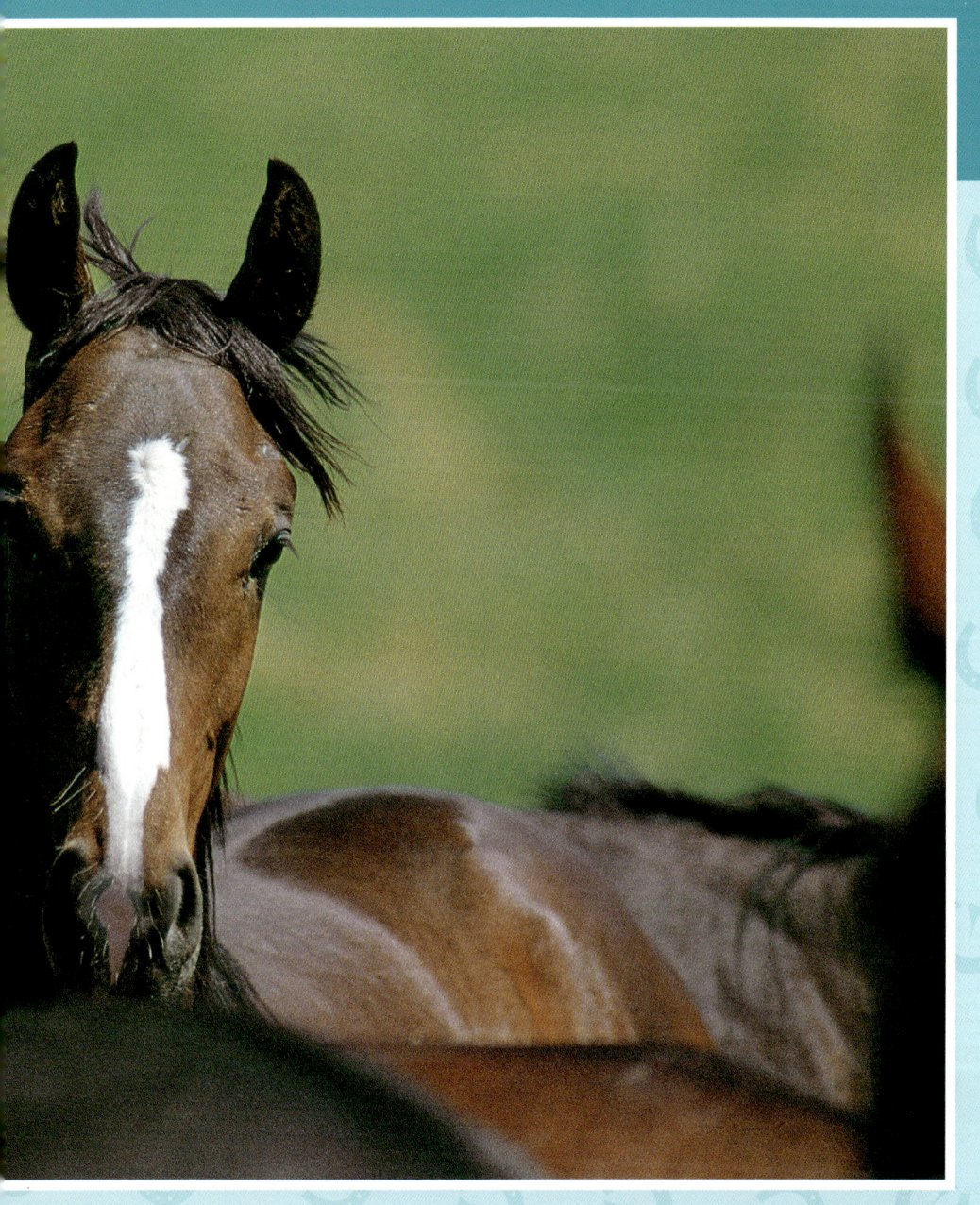

Rediscovering home and natural remedies

Thousands of years before our era, humans discovered the healing powers of nature and used them for their health. The great knowledge of the Native Americans and of Australia's and New Zealand's aborigines is valid to this day, but unfortunately has not been preserved completely. The Egyptians, Greeks and Romans laid the foundations of phytotherapy (herbal medicine), and their experience still benefits us even now. Herbal medicine enjoys great popularity once again, and tried and tested home remedies from the kitchen and the garden form part of our nutrition and health plans. Even in prehistoric times, people derived strength for their immune system from the pharmacy of nature. We too would do well to preserve and apply this knowledge in order to maintain our own health and that of our animals.

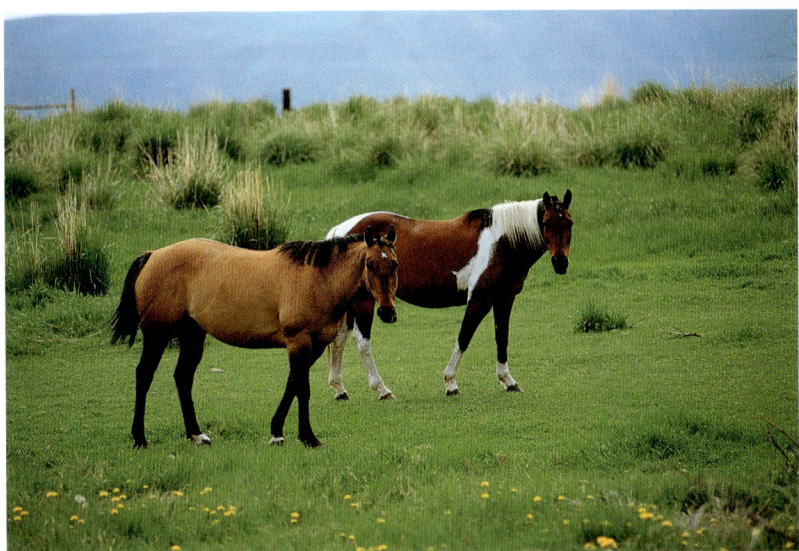

Healthy horses with help from nature

When building the Egyptian pyramids, the slaves strengthened their immune system with fresh garlic and fruit juice, mixed with *Aloe vera*. More than 6,000 years ago, the Chinese made up a brew from ginseng roots and aloe leaves to prevent health problems. Factors that activate self-recovery forces in humans can also strengthen a horse's vitality and health to an advanced age. This book is designed to help you become familiar with natural home and herbal remedies and use them correctly. The focus should be on preventive measures designed to maintain the health of your horse. Appropriate care, movement and a balanced diet are the prerequisites for a healthy horse. With natural remedies and proper attention we can support the vet's work, make good use of time until the vet arrives and speed up the healing process. Medicinal herbs can cure mild complaints, and help the horse to regain fitness more quickly after a long and serious illness. This book is not meant to be a substitute for the vet or natural health practitioner: first and foremost, its purpose is to contribute to disease prevention by utilising the healing powers of nature, building up the resistance of our horses and maintaining their long-term health.

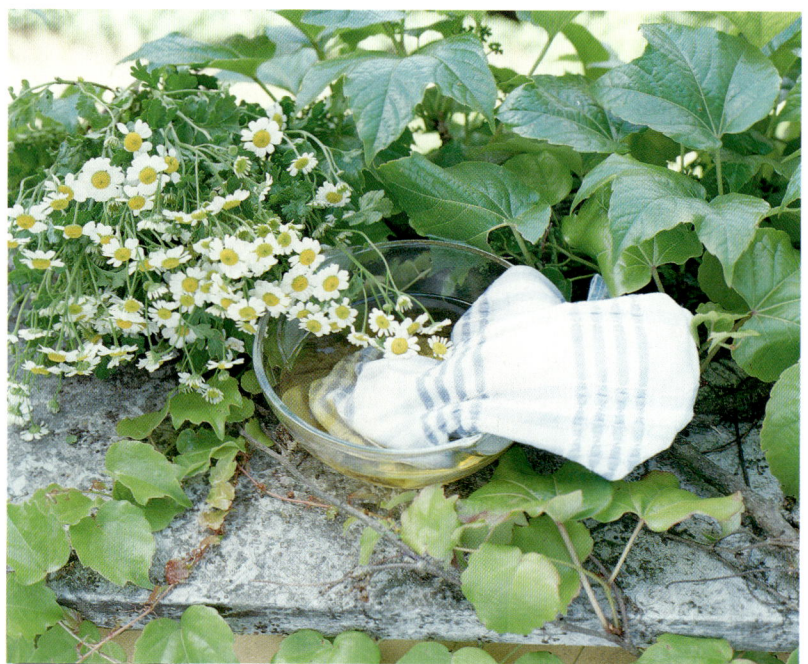

Symptoms	Remedies
Age-related ailments	Algae **15**, Birch leaves **26**, Buckwheat **32,** Cider vinegar **40**, Comfrey **44**, Garlic **69**, Green tea **81**, Hawthorn **84,** Mistletoe **112**, Nettle **117**, Yoghurt **158**
Cardiovascular system	Coneflower **46**, Dandelion **48**, Garlic **69**, Ginseng **75**, Green tea **81**, Hawthorn **84,** Hay flowers **86**, Mistletoe **112**, Nettle **117**, Peppermint **125**, Rosemary **133**, Marian thistle **137**, Water **148**
Colic	Anise–fennel–caraway mix **35, 175**, Chamomile **38**, Comfrey **44**, Liquorice **104**, Marsh mallow **108**, Valerian **145**
Cough/bronchitis	Anise **19**, Chamomile **38**, Coltsfoot **42**, Comfrey **44**, Coneflower **46**, Elderberry **53**, Fennel **61**, Garlic **69**, Iceland moss **94**, Lime blossom **100**, Liquorice **104**, Marsh mallow **108**, Rosehip **131**, Sage **135**, Thyme **143,** Yarrow **156**
Eczema/skin problems	Aloe vera **17**, Black caraway **27**, Chamomile **38**, Cider vinegar **40**, Dandelion **48**, Garlic **69**, Horsetail **65**, Marsh mallow **108**, Meadowsweet **110**, Nettle **117**, Rosehip **131**
Eye inflammation	Buckwheat **32,** Eyebright **59**
Fatigue	Arnica **21**, Coneflower **46**, Garlic **69**, Nettle **117**, Rosehip **131**, Valerian **145**
Fertility disorders	Anise **19**, Fenugreek **63**, Ginseng **75**, Liquorice **104,** Monk's pepper **114**, Peppermint **125**, Raspberry **129**
Fungal infection	Black caraway **27**, Cider vinegar **40**, Coneflower **46**, Garlic **69**, Grapefruit seed extract **79**, Lavender **98**, Marigold **106**, Tea tree oil **141**
General lowered immunity	Cider vinegar **40**, Coneflower **46**, Fungi **66**, Garlic **69**, Ginseng **75**, Green tea **81**, Honey **88**, Nettle **117**, Water **148**
Hooves	Buckwheat **32**, Comfrey **44**, Hawthorn **84**, Horsetail **65**, Lavender **98**, Nettle **117**, Rosehip **131**
Immune system	Coneflower **46,** Garlic **69**, Ginseng **75**, Goosegrass **77**, Green tea **81**, Horsetail **65**, Iceland moss **94**, Marigold **106**, Nettle **117**, Rosehip **131**, Rosemary **133**
Inflammations	Arnica **21**, Black caraway **27**, Cabbage leaves **150**, Chamomile **38**, Comfrey **44**, Coneflower **46**, Goosegrass **77**, Grapefruit seed extract **79**, Hawthorn **84**, Horsetail **65**, Lavender **98**, Marsh mallow **108**, Nettle **117**, Meadowsweet **110**, Willow bark **152**
Laminitis	Comfrey **44**, Dandelion **48**, Garlic **69**, Goosegrass **77**, Hawthorn **84**, Nettle **117**,Yarrow **156**
Metabolism	Birch leaves **26**, Cider vinegar **40**, Dandelion **48**, Devil's claw **50**, Garlic **69**, Goosegrass **77**, Nettle **117**
Milk deficiency	Anise **19**, Buckwheat **32**, Carrots **36**, Fennel **61**, Linseed **102**, Marsh mallow **108**, Nettle **117**
Mouth/teeth	Chamomile **38**, Cider vinegar **40**, Green tea **81**, Sage **135**, Tea tree oil **141**

Symptoms	Remedies
Mud fever	Comfrey **44**, Coneflower **46**, Goosegrass **77**
Musculoskeletal system	Buckwheat **32**, Chamomile **38**, Cider vinegar **40**, Comfrey **44**, Dandelion **48**, Devil's claw **50**, Garlic **69**, Ginger **71**, Goosegrass **77**, Green tea **81**, Hawthorn **84**, Hay flowers **86**, Marigold **106**, Meadowsweet **110**, Mistletoe **112**, Nettle **117**, Rosemary **133**, Water **148**, Willow bark **152**
Nervous system/the mind	Black caraway **27**, Chamomile **38**, Elderberry **53**, Fungi **00**, Ginseng **75**, Honey **88**, Hops **90**, Lavender **98**, Rosemary **133**, St. John's wort **139**, Valerian **145**
Oedema	Chamomile **38**, Cider vinegar **40**, Comfrey **44**, Dandelion **48**, Hawthorn **84**, Horsetail **65**, Nettle **117**
Rheumatism	Algae **15**, Arnica **21**, Chamomile **38**, Cider vinegar **40**, Comfrey **44**, Dandelion **48**, Goosegrass **77**, Lavender **98**, Marigold **106**, Meadowsweet **110**, Nettle **117**, Rosemary **133**, Marian thistle **137**, Tea tree oil **141**, Yarrow **156**
Stomach/bowel	Anise **19**, Caraway **34**, Chamomile **38**, Elderberry **53**, Fennel **61**, Fenugreek **63**, Ginger **71**, Honey **88**, Liquorice **104**, Marsh mallow **108**, Meadowsweet **110**, Peppermint **125**, Valerian **145**, Willow bark **152**, Yoghurt **158**
Warts	Dandelion **48**, Garlic **69**, Marigold **106**, Nettle **117**, Rosehip **131**

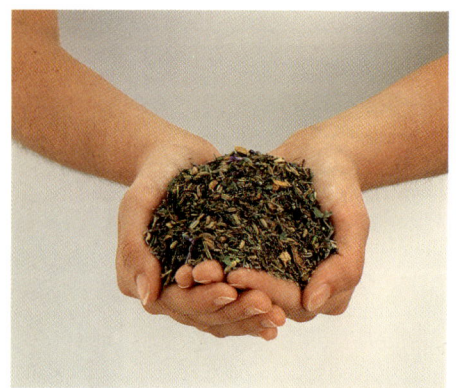

The right application and dosage

Herbs

Properly cared-for horses usually have a good instinct, and on a herb-rich meadow often seek out the plants they need at the time. When riding out, however, you should never let your horse eat indiscriminately since it's easy to get hold of poisonous plants this way.

But since our pastures are not such herb-rich meadows, and since many horses go out only for a few hours a day, we need to find the right herbs for them ourselves.

Herbs, especially fresh plants, do not have to be given in precise doses. Our feeding recommendations are only general guidelines. Ponies can be given a little less than full-sized horses, but the differences are insignificant. You can give your horse two to three handfuls of fresh herbs or around

30 g dried herbs daily. When feeding with herbal mixtures, give 10 g of each herb. Fresh herbs should be chopped up coarsely and mixed into the food. Ready-made commercial herbal mixtures can be given according to the user instructions. All the herbs described in this book are available from pharmacies. They can also make up mixtures for you. Popular medicinal herbs can be purchased from the chemist or health food shops. You can grow some fresh herbs yourself or buy them from the greengrocer.

Tea and infusions

Tea

Pour nearly boiling water (around 500 ml) over 30 g dried or 75–100 g fresh herbs and let the tea brew for 10–15 minutes. After 15 minutes, once it has cooled down and is lukewarm, you can pour the tea with the herbs over food or give it to your horse to drink as it is.

Decoction

Decoctions are suitable for external application, for example as a poultice or for washing wounds. Prepare a tea from fresh or dried herbs as described above. After 15 minutes, the herbs are filtered out with a strainer and the tea used as a decoction.

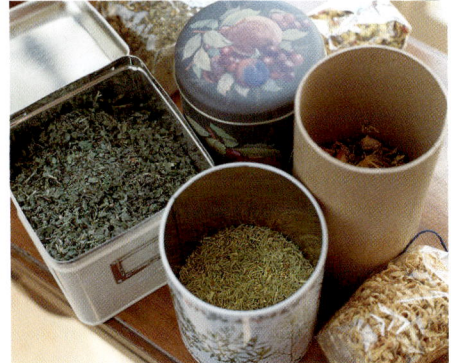

Compress

Compresses are useful for the treatment of eye inflammations or small wounds. Apply the tea or decoction to a sterile lint compress and hold it against the affected site, or in the event of a leg injury, attach it with a bandage.

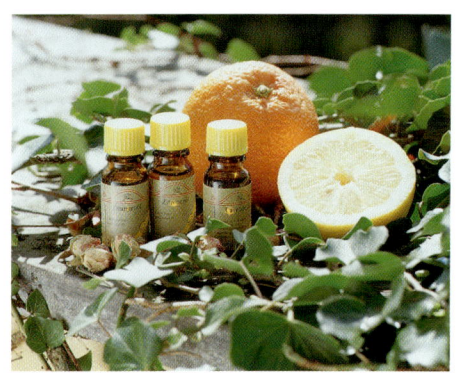

Essential oils

Without detailed knowledge, you should use essential oils only for inhaling and for external application. For massage, compresses and washing, dilute them with carrier oils, for example avocado oil or water.

For inhalation, place hay in a bucket, drizzle 10–15 drops of oil over the hay and pour hot water over it. For blunt injuries, contusions or strained muscles, the oil can be applied in pure form.

Essential oils reach the body through the skin. When the aromatic molecules evaporate, they flow into the horse's nose and pass on information to parts of the brain. This has a positive effect on the horse's well-being.

Important essential oils for horses are contained in garlic, frankincense, chamomile, peppermint, lavender and tea tree. In many cases, aromatherapy practitioners can achieve excellent results when treating diseases.

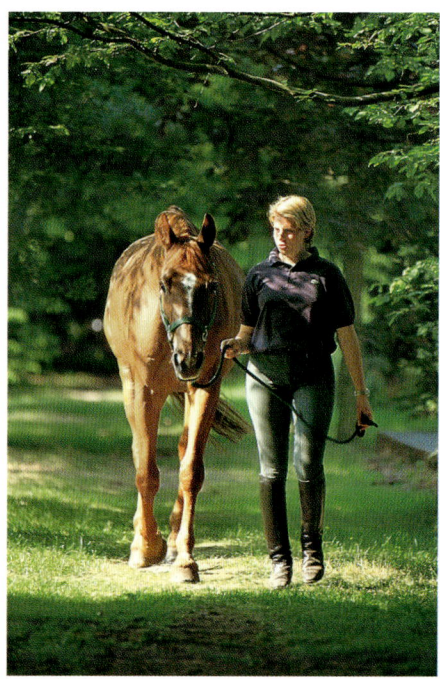

The limits of self-treatment

Every horse owner and rider who spends a great deal of time with horses knows the language of his or her own animals. When I enter the stable, I can see at once whether my four-legged friends are feeling well. In the event of any kind of serious medical complaint, I contact the vet and discuss how I can effectively support his professional treatment. Care is required when planning to participate in tournaments: new rules regarding medication have been in force since 28 April 2010. For example, arnica is prohibited in competitions, and a waiting period of at least two days must be maintained for lavender, liquorice, thyme, devil's claw and eucalyptus. A list of prohibited substances and those with waiting periods, and a listing of permitted substances, can be found here: http://www.fei.org/fei/cleansport/ad-h/prohibited-list (accessed Sept 2015).

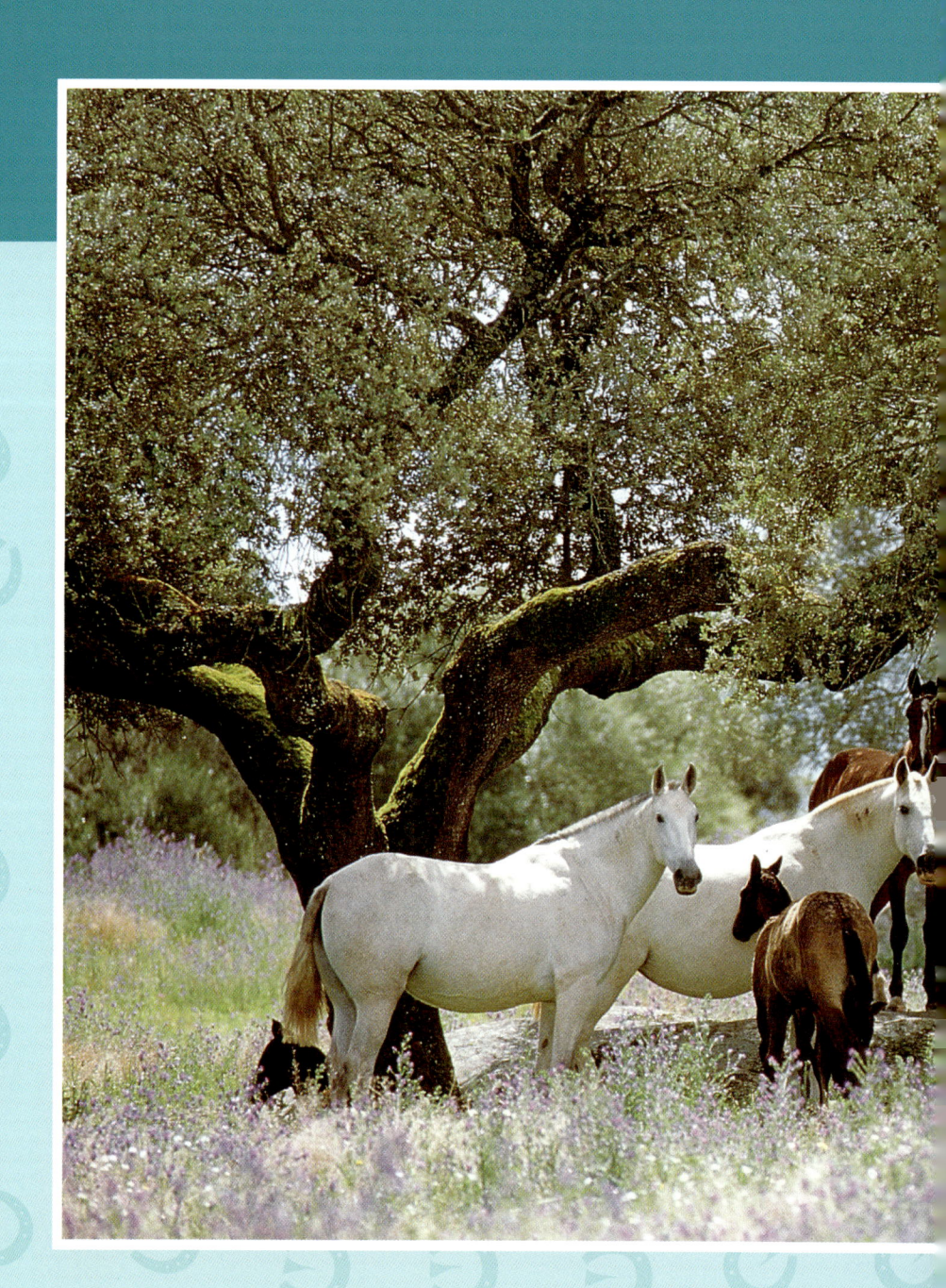

Home and natural remedies from a to z

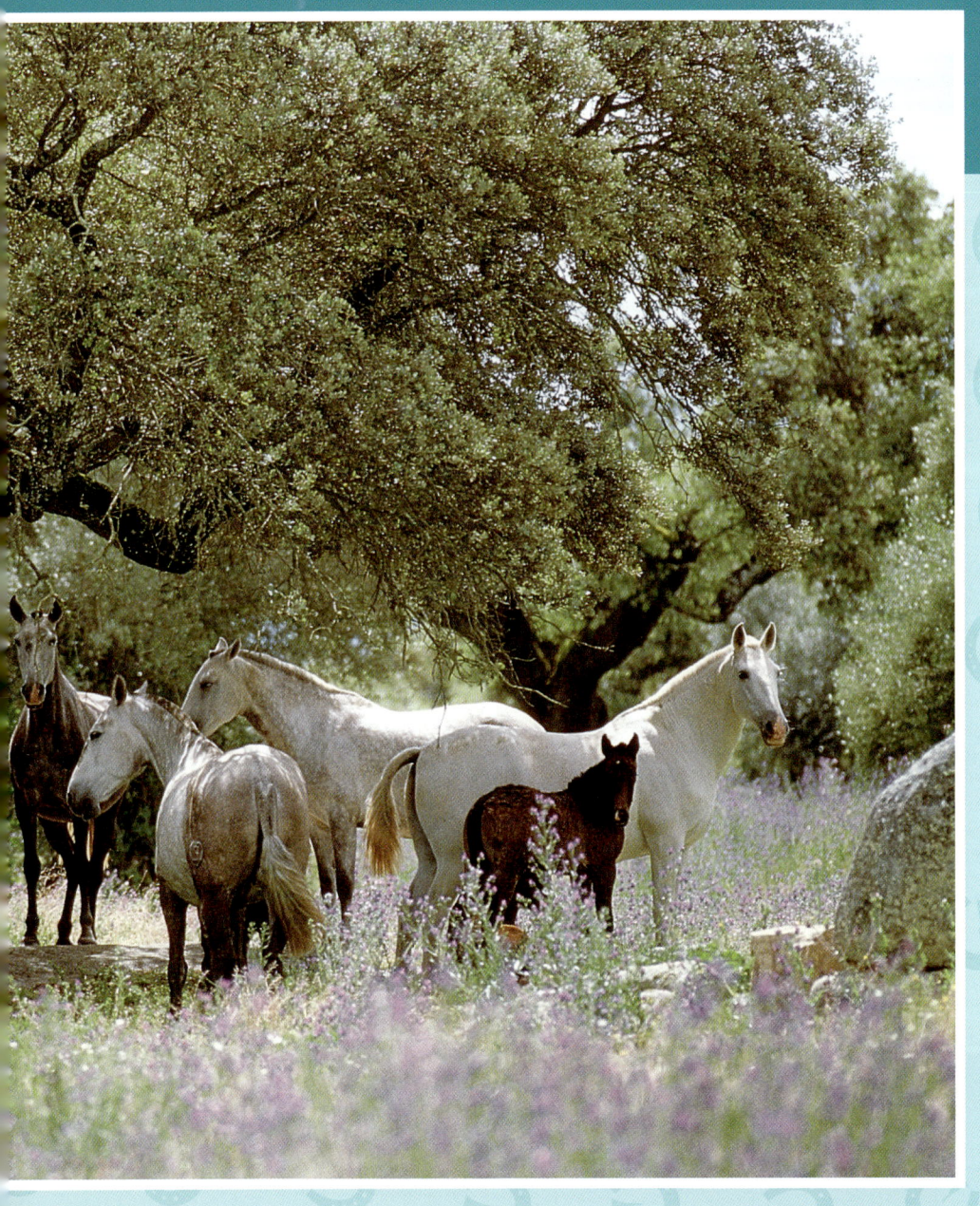

Algae

The origins

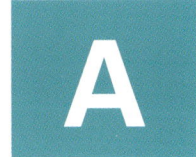

Algae have been around for aeons. They are considered to be plants, even though they don't have any flowers, leaves or roots. Algae are divided into two large groups: saltwater and freshwater algae. All algae have two things in common: they are great survivors, and have an important influence on our climate. Over 20,000 species of algae exist on our planet. In China and Japan, algae have been among the most important food supplements for centuries. While saltwater algae are prized for their high iodine content, freshwater algae are preferred in some thyroid disorders. The latter, for example Chlorella, are especially suitable for managed cultivation and are greatly valued worldwide.

> Detoxifying and body-cleansing effect
> For more stamina and endurance
> Against summer eczema
> For mouth inflammations

IN USE

We can plant many medicinal plants in our own garden, but the algae from the goldfish pond are not suitable for feeding to horses. Here we need to rely on commercial products. Many food or herbal mixtures for horses contain algae.

> DOSAGE

Chlorella can be purchased as a powder or in tablet form. It is easy to prepare the right dosage and give it to the horse with apples, carrots or other treats. The powder is simply sprinkled over food.

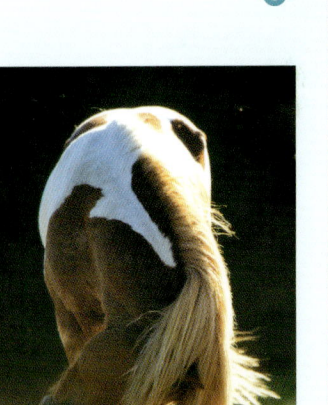

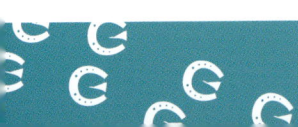

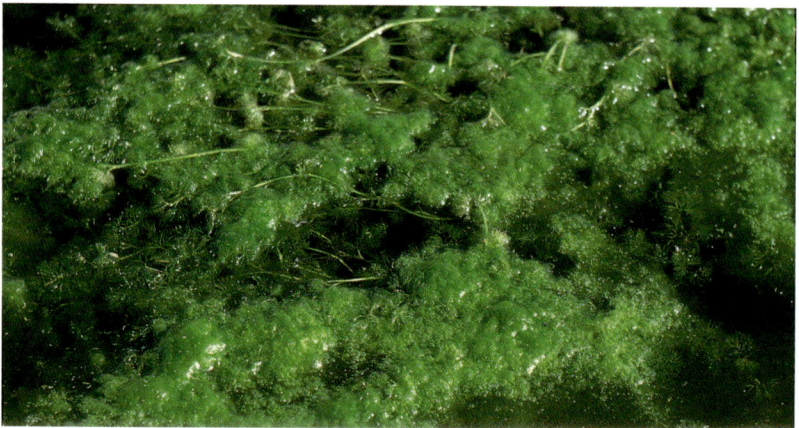

TIP FOR THE RIDER

Algae in powder or tablet form help both horse and rider

Medicinal properties

One of the best known and most thoroughly studied algae is Chlorella. Chlorella contains more chlorophyll than any other living organism, and has a powerful blood- and body-cleansing effect. It contains unsaturated fatty acids, 12 vitamins including the entire vitamin B complex and important minerals and trace elements. The chemical structure of the chlorophyll is almost identical to that of haemoglobin in the blood. Chlorella has an oxygen-enriching effect on the blood. Numerous scientific studies have shown its positive effect on the digestive system, on cholesterol levels and on the immune system. In particular, it has a notable role in binding environmental pollutants, a property that is helpful in allergies, rheumatism, atopic dermatitis and many other medical conditions. Chlorella promotes good eyesight and may have a preventive effect against cancer.

Algae for horses

Giving algae to horses is nothing new; it is common to add algae to the herb and mineral food mixture given to horses suffering from eczema. Pastures have not been herbal meadows for a long time. Therefore, the vitamins and vital substances contained in algae are an excellent means of enriching equine nutrition. Algae help with nearly all complaints that your horse may have. They have a powerful detoxifying effect on all organs and your horse will gain in stamina and endurance. Furthermore, giving algae helps with chronic inflammations of the tendons, ligaments, joints and the respiratory tract. Algae extracts promote the regeneration of the cell's surface, thus counteracting inflammation.

Aloe vera   *Aloe vera*

> For treating wounds and scars
> For eczema and burns
> For care of mane and tail

The origins

The original home of the aloes is likely to have been the region around the Mediterranean, but their health-giving qualities are also very familiar to the Chinese. Aloe vera was first mentioned in old Egyptian writings 3,500 years ago. Nefertiti and Cleopatra had a fondness for using the milk of this plant in their body care. Great armies in history used aloe on their long marches as protection against skin rash and to heal battle wounds. The missionaries in South America, Mexico and Africa knew a great deal about this natural remedy in treating their patients at their infirmaries.

At the end of the Second World War, the aloe helped many Japanese who had been exposed to the burning effects of the atom bombs. With Aloe vera, wounds heal very quickly and without scars.

Medicinal properties

Aloe vera is used first and foremost as an external remedy. The concentrated juice from the leaves is processed into gels, oils and ointments. The numerous

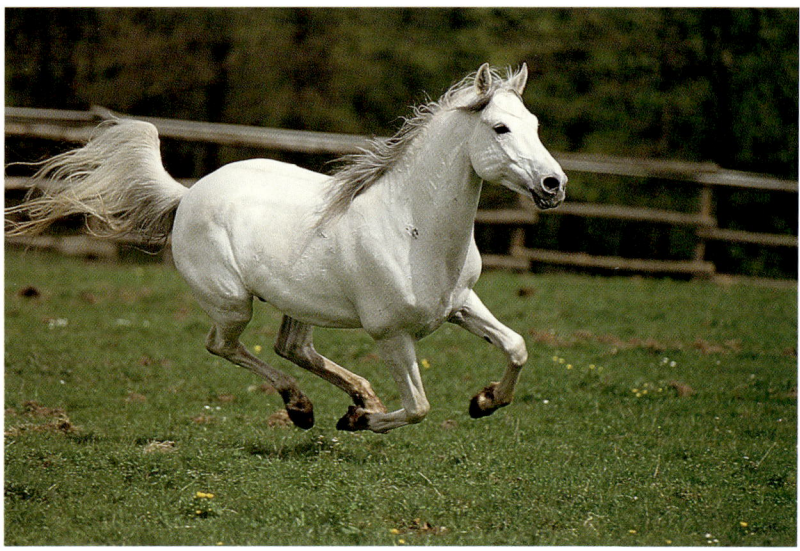

Horses with a light-coloured coat are most prone to sunburn.

ingredients such as vitamins, especially the B group, mucilage, bitter substances, minerals and amino acids have a strong positive effect on the body's immune system and regenerate the skin. Especially in the case of burns and radiation damage, aloe is an important natural remedy. The unprocessed juice of the plant must not be taken internally, since it has a strong laxative effect. In the case of juice, drops and other preparations, the laxative substance is removed.

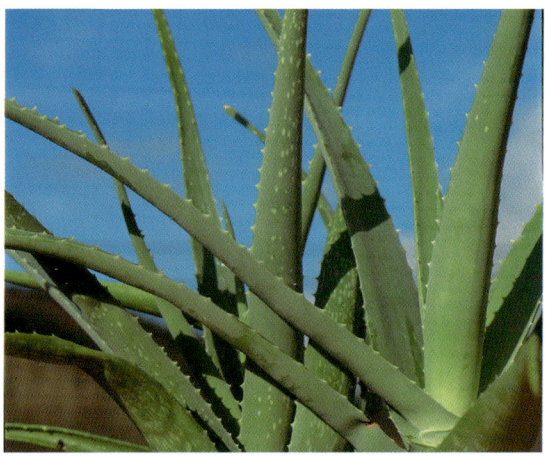

Aloe vera for horses

The external application of Aloe vera is a tried and tested method in veterinary medicine, especially in horses. The juice is a decongestant, pain-relieving, healing and astringent substance. Amazing success can be achieved in the treatment of wounds and scars. Aloe vera helps in eczema, burns and sunburn, which horses too suffer from. Aloe vera is also suitable for bathing fresh wounds and for treating a matted, unkempt coat.

IN USE

Fresh Aloe vera juice from a cut leaf is the quickest and simplest option. The leaves stay fresh for several days in the refrigerator. However, the active agent is also available as a powder, gel, ointment and lotion. Some body lotions contain Aloe vera.

> USED EXTERNALLY

I use Aloe vera body lotion to wash small wounds and occasionally to clean the hooves thoroughly; in the summer I use it to wash all the horses and groom the tail and mane. Our 'free-running horses' especially, are groomed with Aloe vera. Mixed with fruit vinegar, it is an outstanding preparation against itches of all kinds.

Anise   *Pimpinella anisum*

> Soothes the respiratory tract
> Soothes the gastrointestinal system
> Promotes oestrus

The origins

Anise as a spice came originally from Egypt. Nowadays it is cultivated in almost all warm climates. It is very popular as a spice in many dishes, drinks and especially in pastry. The dried seeds are also used widely as a medicinal substance. Anise mixed with other herbs is a popular product.

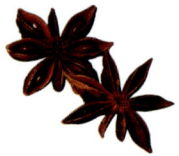

Medicinal properties

Anise is given internally and externally. It acts as an expectorant for a congested respiratory tract, and as an antispasmodic and soothes the gastrointestinal tract. Anise is useful for persistent cough and for digestive disorders, and is especially recommended for babies and toddlers due to its mild effect.

IN USE

> USED INTERNALLY

Application in horses is very simple, since most horses like the flavour of anise. In particular, they are keen on tea mixtures made from the seeds or blossoms. However, it is also possible to add the anise seeds to food (a handful per day). Anise is added to most herbal or food mixtures for horses.

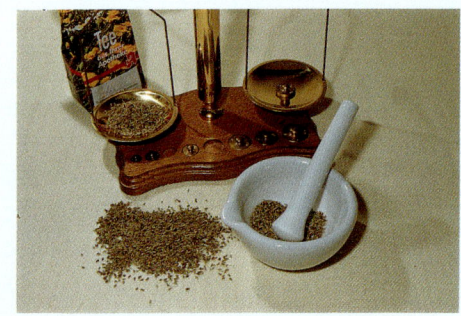

Given regularly, anise has a positive effect on the respiratory tract and calms the digestive system, which many horses benefit from especially during the cold part of the year.

> USED EXTERNALLY

In case of lice, mites or other external parasites, try a daily wash (strong tea or decoction) or apply anise oil.

Anise for horses

In horses too, anise is especially valued for soothing the respiratory tract. Fresh infections and protracted or chronic bronchitis can benefit from anise. In case of colic and gastrointestinal irritation, anise can always be added to other treatments.

Anise is said to have an oestrus-promoting effect, which as a breeder you could make good use of.

Externally, the essential oil of anise can be used to combat lice and mange mites.

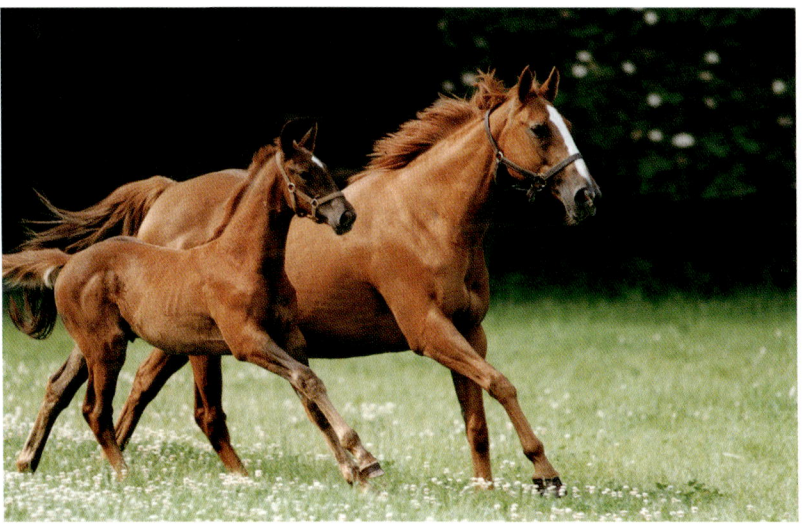

Anise is interesting for breeders, because it is said to have an oestrus-promoting effect.

Arnica   *Arnica montana*

The origins

The name arnica first appears in the 14th century, although its use can be traced back to the early Middle Ages. The plant was used externally and internally against many complaints and ailments.

> For immediate use in injuries
> For overstrained legs
> For contusions

The part mainly used for medicinal purposes is the flowers, which are harvested in July.

The plant grows in poor grasslands, especially at high altitudes and on acid soils. Unfortunately it has become quite rare. In some places it is completely protected, elsewhere only the roots may not be dug up.

Medicinal properties

The active ingredients in arnica are the essential oil, resins, tannins, bitter substances, wax, malic acid and silicic acid. It has an astringent, anti-inflammatory, scar-forming and wound-healing effect. Arnica can be used internally and externally. It strengthens the immune system by activating the white blood cells, thus protecting against bacterial infections.

IN USE

> USED INTERNALLY

Only in homeopathic dilution on sugar or bread. Use immediately after injury or shock.

> USED EXTERNALLY

When used externally as an ointment or tincture, arnica shows excellent effects in contusions, wounds, muscle pain, over-exertion and blunt injuries. Arnica washes for cooling the horse's legs also have proven benefits, when around 5 ml arnica is mixed with 2 l water.

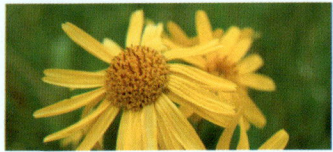

Arnica for horses

Arnica belongs in every medicine cabinet and every stable. It is especially helpful when immediately on hand to deal with injuries.

For hot, over-strained legs, dilute arnica with water and wash the legs.

For blunt injuries up to the knee, place the leg in a bucket and add arnica diluted with water. Once the horse realises how pleasant the effect is, it will usually remain standing patiently. Talking to the horse encouragingly and offering it carrots can sweeten the waiting time. As a herb or tincture, arnica should be used only externally. For highly effective internal administration to treat all kinds of injuries, natural healing practitioners recommend that arnica should be given only in homeopathic dilutions, but always consult your vet.

Arnica is a boon for over-strained legs.

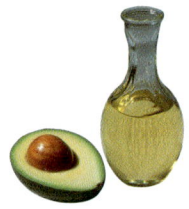

Avocado   *Persea americana*

The origins

The avocado is a member of the laurel family and comes from Central America. It is grown as a cultivated crop in all tropical regions. As a vegetable, it is conquering the European market with ever increasing success. The fragrant flowers are not used for medicinal purposes; instead, we eat the pear-shaped fruit of this exotic plant.

> Helps with coat problems, small wounds and scaly skin
> Helps with summer eczema
> Suitable as a carrier oil for many active substances

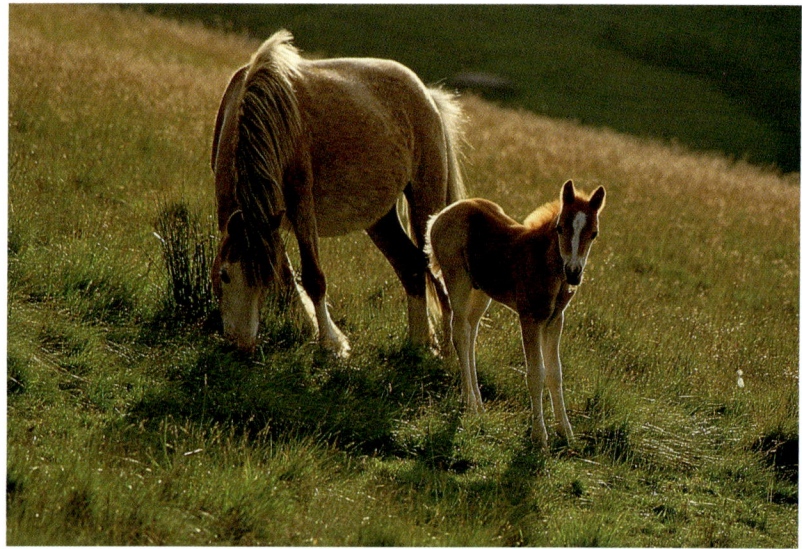

Avocado oil alleviates itching caused by summer eczema.

Medicinal properties

The flesh of the avocado fruit is rich in fatty substances, offering a tasty variation in our kitchen. Avocados are very nutritious and easily digestible. The main product derived from avocados is cooking oil. It is very similar to olive oil and contains vitamins E, A and B, amino acids, lecithin and antibiotic substances. Medically, it is used to treat eczema, and scaly, dry and highly sensitive skin. Avocado oil is very well tolerated and does not irritate the skin and mucosal tissue.

IN USE

A few years ago, two of my grazing horses suffered from an unexplainable itch. The vet could not work out the cause, either. After giving it some thought, I first washed the affected areas with a mixture of cider vinegar and a commercial washing lotion containing aloe, yucca and coconut oil. Then I mixed avocado oil, camphor oil and a cream containing evening primrose oil in a pot and rubbed the mixture into my horses' skin every day. The skin improved, the itch subsided and the coat grew back all shiny. I have also tried this formulation on my goat Rosi. Unfortunately, she is not as keen and amenable as the horses, but the skin problems are improving.

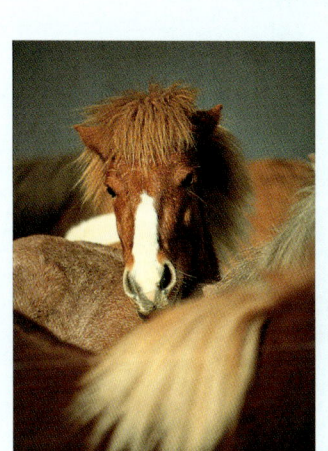

> AVAILABILITY

You can buy avocado oil in health food stores or at the chemist.

> DOSAGE

Apply as needed several times a day, either straight or mixed with other remedies.

Avocado for horses

I have achieved very good results with avocado oil in the treatment of skin and coat problems, for example summer eczema. It is also extraordinarily suitable as a carrier oil for all substances that have to be applied to wounds and to scaly or cracked skin. Whenever remedies such as tea tree oil, camphor or eucalyptus seem too strong on their own, add some avocado oil. It makes the skin soft, has a calming effect, improves wound healing and does not irritate the skin.

The avocado fruit may be suitable as a food supplement for thin or malnourished horses. So far, I have not yet tried it with my horses.

B

Birch leaves *Betulae folium*

The origins

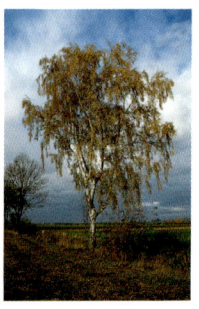

In Germanic traditions, the birch had a special role as a charm. It was believed that anyone whipped with a birch twig before sunrise on Easter Sunday, would be blessed with good health for the whole year. During Walpurgis night, the witches rode birch broomsticks up to the Blocksberg peak.

But the birch has retained its magic even without the dance of the witches. In earlier times, the juice of young birch trees was made into a hair tonic and the bark used to treat wounds.

This well-loved tree grows in humid soils almost everywhere in the world. Today the leaves are used medicinally, as already recommended by Hildegard of Bingen. Birch leaves are easy to obtain and are usually brewed into a tea.

> For cleansing the blood
> For older and weaker horses
> Against fluid retention

Medicinal properties

Birch leaves contain flavonoids, tannins and saponins, and are valued for their regulating effect on the body's fluid balance. They are used to increase urine production and to treat disorders in which elevated urine quantities are desirable, for example to prevent kidney stones. Birch leaves are also recommended for cleansing the blood and for skin blemishes.

Teas for rheumatism and metabolic conditions contain birch leaves as a useful and efficacious ingredient. Medicinally, one uses the young leaves of the two commonly occurring birch species, those of the silver birch and of the downy birch.

TIP FOR THE RIDER

Birch leaves can be used to enrich salads, soups and stews.

IN USE

> USED INTERNALLY

It is recommended to brew a tea and pour it over food, or to sprinkle individual leaves over it. Birch leaves are available from the pharmacy, or can be picked from the tree.

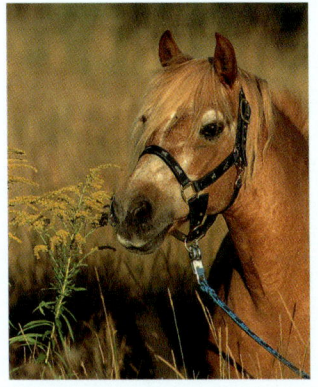

The leaves should be picked in the spring, dried and kept in tightly-closed containers.

> DOSAGE

You can add around 50 g birch leaves to food daily, or make a tea from the leaves and pour it over food.

Birch leaves for horses

In older or weak horses, birch leaves can be used as a general blood cleansing course of treatment. For horses who tend to retain fluids, a condition known as oedema, regular administration of birch leaves or birch tea can enrich food. If the vet finds that your horse has a kidney or bladder disorder, ask him or her whether you could support the treatment with birch leaves.

Herbal mixtures for horses often contain dried birch leaves.

A TIP FROM THE VET

In cases of oedema, always have your horse's heart and lungs examined by the vet.

Black caraway   *Nigella sativa*

The origins

True black caraway, often called just black caraway, is a plant in the buttercup family. It is unrelated to caraway. Black caraway comes from India, western Asia, southern Europe and especially from North Africa. In the Orient, it has been valued for over 2,000 years as a pepper-like spice and

> Remedy of first choice for allergies
> Inhibits fungal and bacterial growth
> Effective against summer eczema

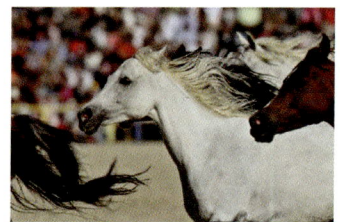

We can thank a valuable Arabian horse for the rediscovery of black caraway in Germany. It suffered from severe asthma attacks, which proved resistant to all veterinary treatments. A physician from Egypt recommended black caraway seed and oil. In Egypt, Arabian horses have been treated with this remedy for thousands of years. The sick horse recovered completely, and from this point black caraway started its success story in Germany.

medicine. Since its flavour is reminiscent of sesame, in Asia and Africa it is sprinkled on various flat breads.

'Black caraway heals every illness – except death'. Based on this saying, this herb has become famous in recent centuries throughout Asia. When the fabled Pharaoh Tutankhamen died over 3,000 years ago, a vial of black caraway oil was placed in his sarcophagus for his life after death. The beautiful Egyptian queen Nefertiti anointed her body with this magical oil. And Hippocrates, the most famous physician in antiquity, used black caraway oil for many complaints.

Medicinal properties

Black caraway oil and seeds are used in natural medicine. Modern Western science has rediscovered the value of this old folk remedy.

Many of the over 100 substances found in black caraway have been investigated. The abundant oil contains around 70% unsaturated fatty acids, fat-associated substances and various vitamins. In particular, the high level of linoleic acid, linolenic acid and nigellone is very helpful in combating allergies. Black caraway is regarded as the most successful natural remedy of the last 10 years. From toddler to adult, anyone can be treated with it over prolonged periods. Even conventional medicine is unanimous in its opinion that it boosts the production of immune system cells, is a strong anti-inflammatory, lowers blood sugar levels and stimulates bone marrow cells. Its curative effects in cases of asthma have been demonstrated at Berlin's Charité hospital. In addition, black caraway is used to treat all kinds of allergies, in cancer therapy, in neurodermatitis, bronchitis, menstrual complaints, depression and inflammation.

TIP FOR THE RIDER

Black caraway oil is available nowadays from equine sport dealers, feed merchants and pharmacies. It should be a high-quality cold pressed oil and 100% unadulterated.

Black caraway for horses

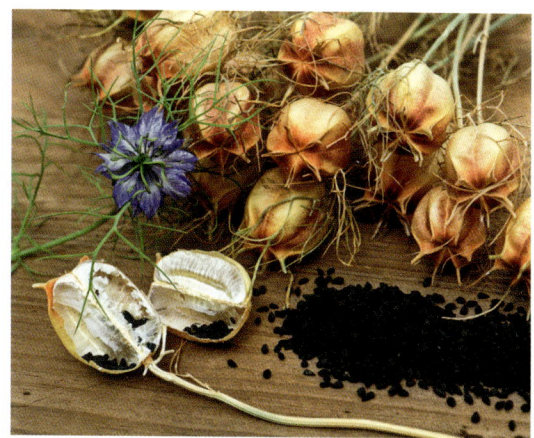

As with humans, the success story continues in the animal kingdom. The oil can be used both internally and externally, and inhibits fungal and bacterial growth. Every form of allergy, for example summer eczema, responds well to this remedy. True black caraway can help to optimise the development of performance, in the event of stress or when changing the diet, to generally boost the immune system and to treat inflammation.

IN USE

> USED EXTERNALLY

Externally, minor wounds, scabby areas, malanders and saddle sores are treated with black caraway oil. For general improvement of the coat, rub the animal with a mixture of a few drops of the oil in water. This results in a silky, sleek coat and also keeps insects away. When applying the oil externally, it is important to make sure that it does not come into contact with the eyes.

> USED INTERNALLY

Egyptian black caraway is especially valued. For internal use, mix it into the regular food. The amount should be stated on the product, or discuss the dosage with your vet.

Average recommended amount: black caraway cake: up to 100 g daily; oil: 12–25 ml daily.

Borage   *Borago officinalis*

Star flower

The origins

It is unknown just how old borage is. It is assumed that it was cultivated in the Middle Ages by the Arabs in Spain. Here and in the rest of Europe, it still occurs frequently in the wild. It grows in waste disposal sites and at roadsides, but due to its positive properties in medicine and cosmetics it is planted commercially across almost the whole of Europe. The fresh leaves and blossoms of borage have a cucumber-like flavour and can be prepared as a salad.

Medicinal properties

The most important ingredients of borage are in the blossoms, leaves and stalks. It contains resins, potassium nitrate, saponins, tannins and mucilage.

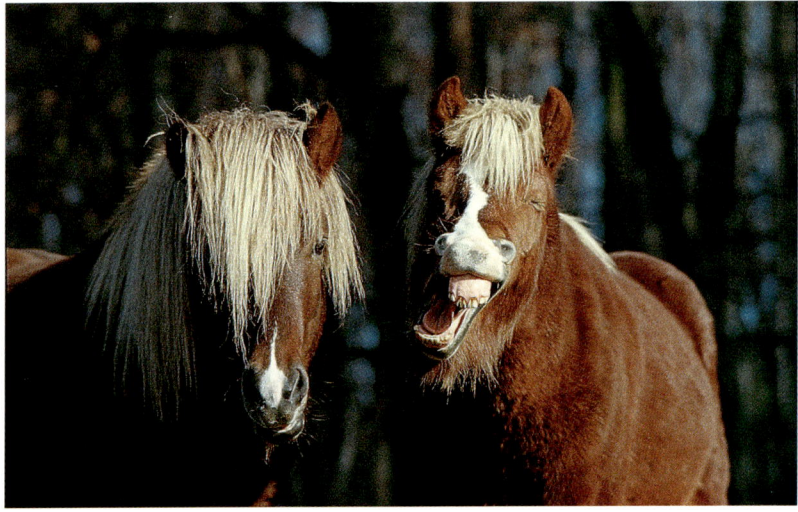

Borage makes tired horses alert.

Taken internally, borage has a sweat-inducing and laxative effect. Borage is a recommended spring remedy and helps in flu, coughs and gout. It can be useful also in excessive perspiration, for example in combination with sage. Used externally, it helps in herpes.

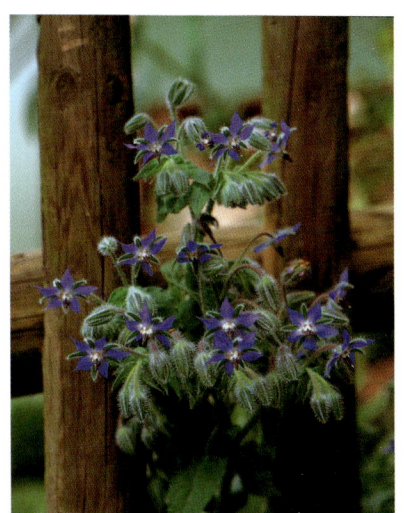

Borage for horses

As a pasture plant, borage strengthens the heart, acts as a diuretic and cleanses the blood. It is a natural performance-boosting remedy in horses. If your horses tend to have swollen legs, borage tea may help: it's worth a try. For long rides or tournaments, borage can be given as a natural, permitted stimulant. Borage, dandelion and nettle tea is a popular spring remedy.

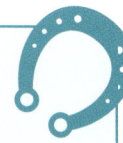

IN USE

Borage can be planted in your garden or in the pasture. Seeds and mixtures are available commercially.

Borage tea can be bought at the pharmacy.

> USED INTERNALLY

A mixture of blossoms and leaves is best suited for tea. Horses like the flavour of the star flower, but other tea mixtures can be added just as well. Borage is also available nowadays in herbal mixtures.

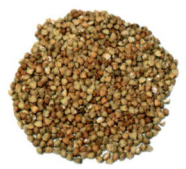

Buckwheat   *Fagopyrum esculentum*

The origins

> Helps in
circulation
disorders
> Effective
against
nosebleeds
> Good for
elderly horses
> Helps in
allergies

Buckwheat originated in central Asia, but was introduced into Europe and North America long ago. In America it is a well-known food, and often replaces wheat flour. Buckwheat pancakes have also become popular in Europe. It plays an ever increasing role in health-conscious cuisine.

These days, many people have an allergic reaction to wheat and wheat flour. Unfortunately, this is seen more and more in babies and toddlers. Buckwheat products are a good solution: they are tasty and can replace almost all wheat products. Moreover, nowadays buckwheat is grown organically more often than in the case of wheat.

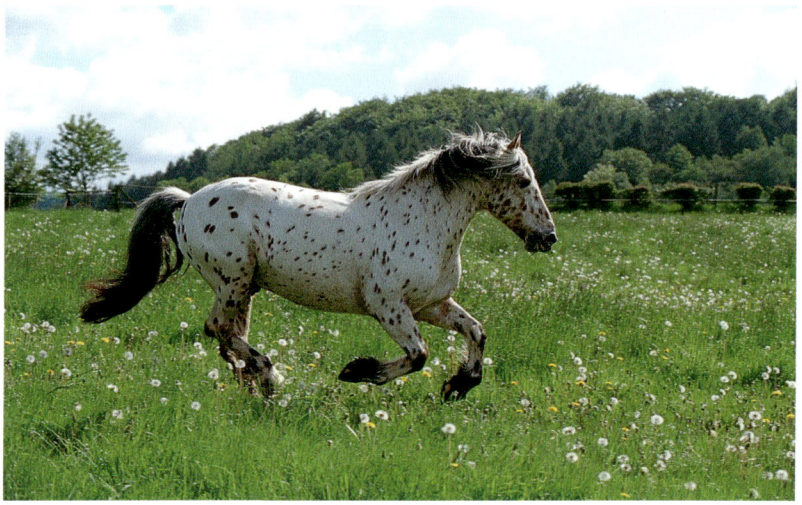

Buckwheat is also used in rheumatism and arthritis.

Medicinal properties

Scientific studies have demonstrated that buckwheat contains many health-promoting substances. It is rich in iron, potassium, calcium, magnesium and trace elements. Rutin, a substance obtained from buckwheat, strengthens the blood vessels and makes them more elastic.

Buckwheat dilates blood vessels and strengthens the fine capillaries. Its antipruritic effect too, helps people who suffer from allergies with their skin problems.

IN USE

Only the dried parts of buckwheat without the roots are utilised as a herb. The seeds are milled like flour and used in the kitchen, for example in pancakes. The plants are collected during the flowering season and dried. If you don't have time to collect the buckwheat yourself, you can buy the dried plant.

> USED INTERNALLY

As with other herbs, mix around 30 g into food. Older horses in particular, should be given buckwheat over a longer period. In the event of summer eczema too, consider giving buckwheat.

Buckwheat for horses

Buckwheat can be helpful in treating all ailments in which better blood circulation is desirable. A tendency to nosebleeds (thoroughbreds especially tend to suffer from these), circulation disorders, rheumatism, arthritis, navicular disease and laminitis can benefit from buckwheat. However, always check first with the vet. Elderly horses should in any event be given buckwheat to stimulate the circulation, ideally in combination with hawthorn and nettle. For horses who have a tendency to allergies, supplement food with buckwheat over a prolonged period.

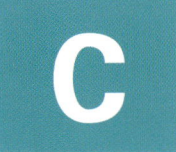

C

Caraway   *Carum carvi*

The origins

The ancient Greeks knew an umbelliferous plant that is likely to have had similar properties to caraway, and later also conferred on caraway its Latin name. Caraway is a spice that occurs in Europe and in the temperate zones of North America and northern Asia. It grows in meadows and pasture and on embankments, and is regarded as a good food plant for animals. In cows and sheep, and certainly also in horses, it promotes milk production.

> Helps when
changing the
diet
> Has a
positive effect
on digestion
> Prevents
colic

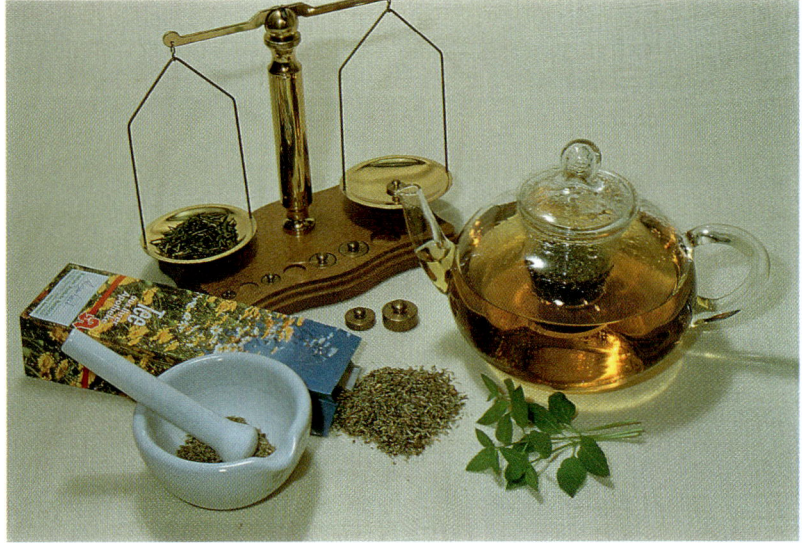

The active ingredients will develop their effect better if you lightly crush caraway, fennel and anise in a mortar.

Medicinal properties

Caraway is a popular spice that makes many dishes more digestible. It contains essential oils, primarily with carvone and limonenes, fatty acids, proteins and tannins. It is known for its antispasmodic effect on the gastrointestinal tract and helps with flatulence or a feeling of fullness, especially after meals that are difficult to digest. Caraway encourages milk production and can regulate menstruation.

Caraway for horses

For horses, the effect of caraway on the digestive system is especially helpful. In addition to other medicinal herbs, horses that tend to suffer from colic can be given a little caraway every day. In the event of illness, stress, a change in the diet and all situations that have a negative effect on digestion, a little caraway will relieve the equine stomach. During the first few days of the grazing season, caraway rebalances the change in dietary composition. Flatulence, which is no more pleasant for a horse than for anyone else, should always be treated with caraway.

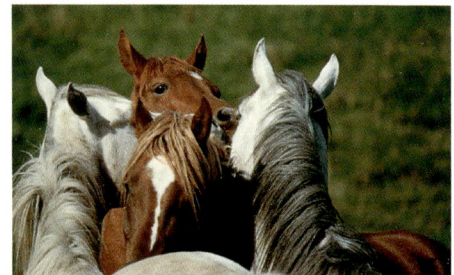

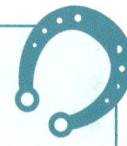

IN USE

> USED INTERNALLY

Caraway can be given to horses in a variety of ways. For our ponies, an anise–fennel–caraway infusion mix is the absolute bestseller.

In case of severe flatulence, try caraway fruits. Freshly ground or crushed, they are mixed into food. One of our horses tends to suffer from bad flatulence when given too much silage. I mash fresh caraway, pour hot water on it, let it stand and then simply pour the infusion with the grains into the manger. Nothing is left behind, not a drop or a single grain.

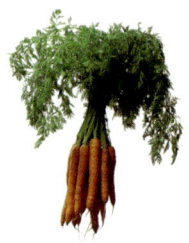

Carrots   *Daucus carota subsp. sativus*

The origins

This yellow–orange root vegetable is one of the most popular in the kitchen, having long ago overcome its image as 'baby food'. In addition to being tasty, the carrot is greatly beneficial to health. It can be grown anywhere and is available in many forms. The easily digestible carrot blends well with many other vegetables, and whether raw or cooked is nutritionally important. Carrots store well and can, therefore, be eaten all year round.

Medicinal properties

The most important and best-known active substance in carrots is carotene, the yellow pigment. It is referred to as provitamin A, and with the help of fat is converted in the body to vitamin A. It has strong medicinal properties that are useful for impaired vision, inflammation, night blindness and tired eyes after long sessions working at the computer screen or reading in poor light. Carrots promote a fresh complexion and are good for the mucous membranes. They are best enjoyed raw or as a salad with a little oil. They should be only very slightly steamed, in order to preserve the vitamins and other important substances.

A TIP FROM THE VET

Fodder carrots don't have the same high beta-carotene content in winter and spring, and one can then resort to powdered products.

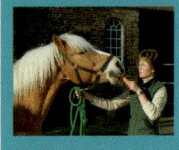

Carrots for horses

Carrots are juicy and add liquid to food. They are a big hit in the stable. Every horse owner, rider or stable hand has pampered, rewarded or even enticed his or her horse with carrots, which horses are very keen to eat. The energy content is about the same as in turnips and 6–7 kg carrots equal 1 kg oats in energy content. In winter especially, carrots are an important supplementary food since other juicy food, for example pasture grass, is in short supply. The fact that carrots are easily digested is also important for horses and they have almost become one of the staple dietary foods.

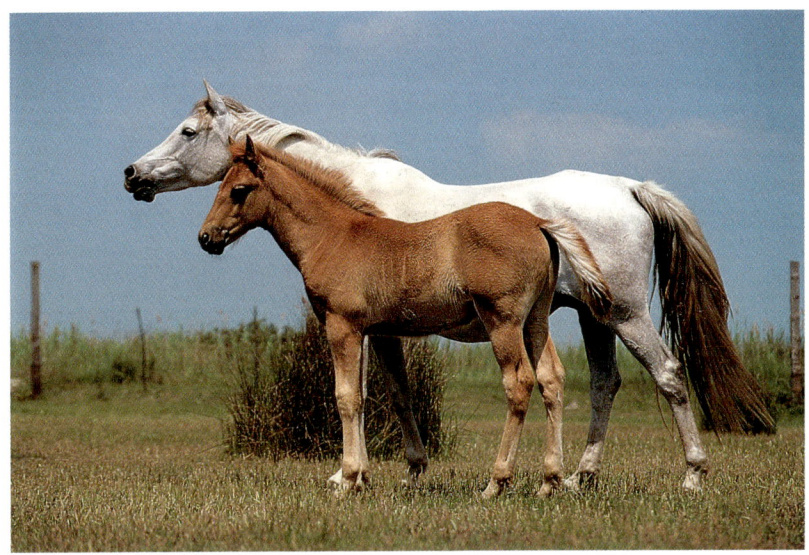

Carrots are especially important for brood mares due to their high carotene content.

IN USE

> USED INTERNALLY

Carrots are available all year round. By all means give your horse several kilograms rather than regarding carrots only as a treat. It is always better to give juicy carrots separately and not simply add them to the concentrated feed. In addition, our horses, when kept in stalls, welcome every in-between meal or snack. It is also beneficial to add a little linseed oil to allow vitamin A to be built up in the body. For old horses who can no longer chew efficiently, rub or crush the carrots with a little oil. Carrots from an organic supplier or your own garden are best for horses too. If this is not possible, wash the carrots before feeding in order to rinse off any pollutants.

Chamomile   *Matricaria chamomilla*

The origins

Many people have childhood memories of being offered chamomile tea and honey when lying ill in bed. Our best-known medicinal plant is a true long-term success, and was used in the past as it is today for many varied purposes.

The chamomile has been a constant for thousands of years, being used from birth to old age.

In ancient Egypt it was the flower of the sun god, and even the Neanderthals surely appreciated its good effects.

Today it is one of the most thoroughly researched medicinal plants, and its benefits are too many to be listed here.

Chamomiles grow almost everywhere, and in the garden one should keep a small corner free for them to thrive in.

Medicinal properties

One reason for the popularity of chamomile is that it has virtually no side-effects. Its medical properties derive from its balanced ingredients: essential oils with the blue substance chamazulene, flavonoids, fatty acids and potassium.

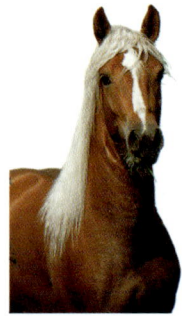

The effect on pain of all kinds is superb, internally and externally. Chamomile is an antiseptic, anti-inflammatory, antispasmodic, sedative and tonic, and is digestion-improving, calming, relaxing and a vasodilator.

It promotes restful sleep and helps babies with colic. The special mucilaginous substances alleviate irritations of the gastrointestinal tract. Furthermore, it has a regulating and calming effect in bilious attacks and menstrual disorders.

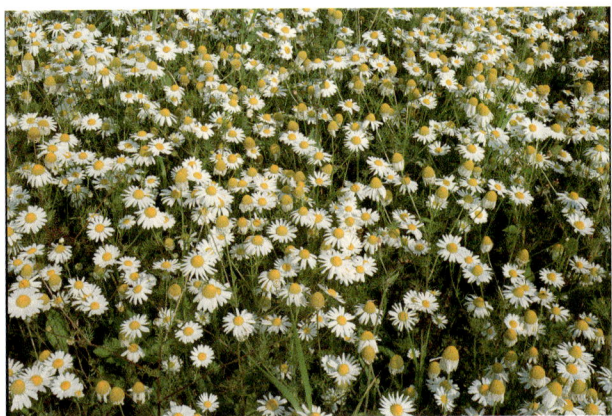

Chamomile for horses

This is a natural remedy that every rider has at home. If your horse suffers from stress, tension or agitation, you can soothe it with chamomile. In colic, and especially after gastrointestinal complaints and other illnesses, warm chamomile tea alleviates cramps and is an anti-inflammatory.

When my vet has to get some fluid into one of our horses, I have chamomile tea ready to add to it.

Wounds of all kinds can be washed out with chamomile. Inflammations, for example mastitis and vaginitis, can be treated with chamomile in addition to veterinary care. I have used chamomile frequently in very fractious and irritable horses as a successful herbal remedy.

A TIP FROM THE VET

Sometimes chamomile is recommended for eye inflammations. Don't follow this advice however: eyebright is much more suitable.

IN USE

> USED INTERNALLY

Tea is the simplest way to take chamomile. Freshly brewed, it can be fed together with the blossoms. You can also sprinkle a handful of dried blossoms over food daily. In the winter especially, my horses get their evening meal served with tea (keep ringing the changes).

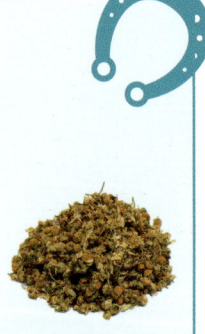

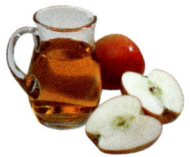

Cider vinegar

The origins

The ancient Egyptians and Babylonians were familiar with it, similarly the Phoenicians, Greeks and Romans, and of course Hildegard of Bingen.

Even before bacteria were known to science, cider vinegar was used for disinfection and as a natural preservative.

> Increases immune resistance
> Regulates the digestive system
> Helps with coughs and bronchitis
> Deters flies and midges
> Helps against tail chafing

Medicinal properties

'An apple a day keeps the doctor away', as the old saying has it. And what apples can do, cider vinegar can do even better. The decisive factor in its extraordinary success is the interaction between more than 30 nutrients that are important for the body. It contains vitamins (A, B, C and E), minerals and trace elements. In addition, it contains quite a high level of pectin. Internally and externally, cider vinegar is germicidal and antibacterial and makes for top fitness.

TIP FOR THE RIDER

Flies are driven away from the stable when troughs, walls and floors are treated frequently with vinegar–water mixtures. Add a little garlic, and the unwanted guests move elsewhere.

Cider vinegar for horses

Cider vinegar has varied uses in horses. Those given it every day are more resistant to all kinds of infection. In particular, the sensitive digestive system of horses is supported and regulated, and unhealthy fermentation processes

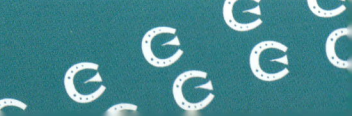

are counteracted. If your horse suffers from coughs or bronchitis, you can give it a mixture of cider vinegar and honey; inhalation can also bring relief. Starting cider vinegar treatment in early spring is an effective way of protecting horses from midges, flies and other biting pests.

In addition to internal use, the coat can be rubbed down with fruit vinegar, especially before riding, since sweating enhances the horse's own odour and attracts flies. Insect bites should be rubbed down at once with straight cider vinegar. This soothes the itch and counteracts any swelling.

After the ride, every horse enjoys being washed down with water and fruit vinegar. Areas prone to pressure, for example the saddle and girth area, are strengthened with cider vinegar, and the tendons and ligaments refreshed after the ride. In horses with persistent tail chafing, you should rub down the dock with cider vinegar and also check the time of the last worming treatment. Cider vinegar therapy can benefit poor hooves and an unkempt coat, and it is also tried and tested for osteoarthritis and rheumatism. Giving cider vinegar internally can also be useful for fungal infections. Horses who tend to refuse any medication can be tricked with fruit vinegar. Mix the medicine, whether as a powder, a gel or a liquid, with fruit vinegar and a little food – most horses will eat the mash without any problems.

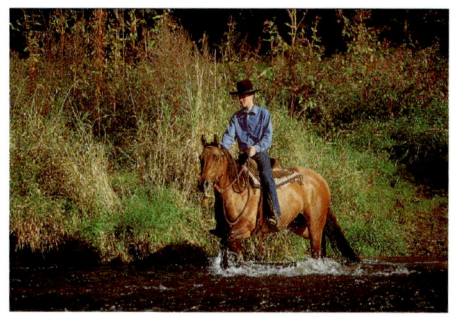

Cider vinegar keeps flies away during summer rides.

IN USE

> USED INTERNALLY

Cider vinegar is taken readily by all horses. Add a daily dash to food, and your horses will stay fit.

Cider vinegar and honey are two home remedies that complement each other superbly, and are equally health-promoting for the rider and the horse. If the horses drink their water from buckets, cider vinegar can also be given with the water.

> USED EXTERNALLY

Externally, cider vinegar can be applied straight or diluted as a poultice, wash or rub-down.

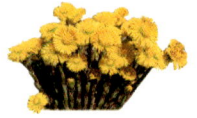

Coltsfoot

Tussilago farfara

The origins

> Acts as an
expectorant
for coughs
> Helps with
sprains
> An anti-
inflammatory
for abscesses

Coltsfoot is one of the first harbingers of spring. Its yellow flowers can be found along verges of roads and in many overgrown places.

Although a useful medicinal plant, often it is decried as a weed. The name Tussilago ('cough repelling') refers to its most important property, its action against coughs and bronchitis. Being highly undemanding, it occurs almost everywhere in Europe, Asia and North Africa. The most important parts for naturopathy are its leaves, but sometimes the flower heads and roots are also utilised.

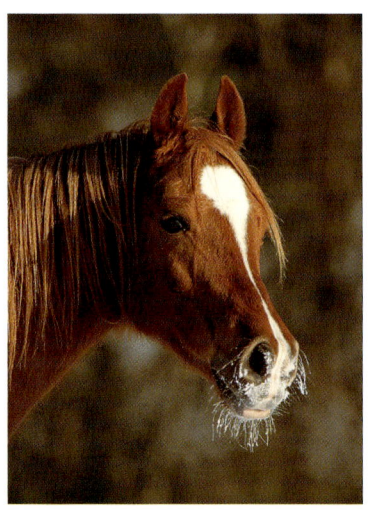

Coltsfoot is a very effective cough remedy.

Wild coltsfoot may contain alkaloids which are highly toxic to the liver, and an alkaloid-free clonal variety, available commercially, was developed in Germany and Austria.

Medicinal properties

The most valuable substances for medicinal use are the mucilage, tannins, gallic acid salts and mineral salts. Coltsfoot leaves promote expectoration, are blood-purifying, sweat-inducing and soothing. Coltsfoot is available as an infusion and as a cough mixture. The pure juice of the plant can also be useful externally. We use its anti-inflammatory properties to treat sprains and wounds, but also for abscesses. Coltsfoot should not be taken during pregnancy and breastfeeding. It is a remedy for acute conditions and is unsuitable for long-term therapy.

Coltsfoot for horses

Coltsfoot for horses is first and foremost a cough remedy. It is contained in juices and powders for coughs and bronchitis. It is used to alleviate irritation caused by inflammation of the oral mucous membranes. Although there is no empirical data, it should not be used in pregnant and suckling mares.

IN USE

Coltsfoot is an ingredient of herbal mixtures for respiratory tract ailments, and is contained in many cough mixtures and powders.

> USED INTERNALLY

Cough medicine used in people can help animals also, and can be given in food or syringed into the mouth. Hop leaf infusion can be given with food.

> Promotes the
musculoskeletal
system of older
horses
> Helps with
sprains,
contusions and
tendon injuries
> Regenerates
tissue

Comfrey   *Symphytum officinale*

Boneset, Knitbone

The origins

The name Symphytum is derived from the Greek word 'symphyein' (to grow together), and in antiquity referred to a number of plants which, like comfrey, were used to heal broken bones. More recent investigations confirm the beneficial properties of comfrey for wounds, fractures and many other complaints. Comfrey is found on river banks, in ditches and in marshy meadows.

Medicinal properties

Comfrey is an excellent tried and tested remedy both in human and in veterinary medicine. Its most important ingredients are alkaloids, mucilage,

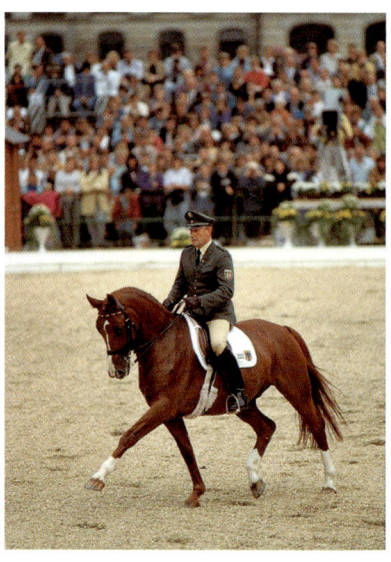
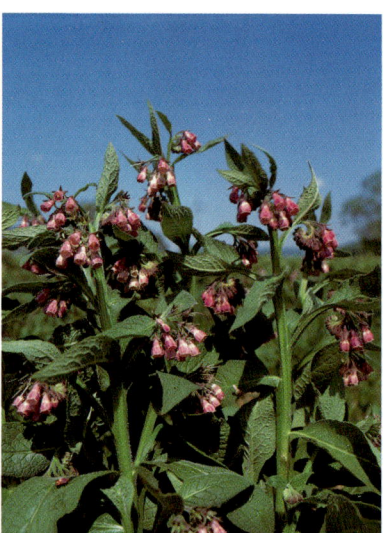

Bones and tendons are at high risk of injury.

tannins, allantoin and essential oil. It has outstanding astringent, anti-inflammatory, emollient, scar-forming, cough-relieving, wound-healing and irritant-soothing properties. Comfrey is used internally and externally for broken bones, sprains, nerve inflammation, burns, psoriasis, skin tumours and other skin conditions, diarrhoea, stomach disorders and angina. The essential oil of comfrey has a powerful antibacterial action.

Comfrey for horses

Almost no other plant is used so widely as a remedy for horses as comfrey. Its ability to rapidly heal bones, connective tissue and even the skin is due to allantoin. Cell division is stimulated and the tissue quickly regenerated. Almost all injuries, such as sprains, contusions, synovial cysts, injured tendons and rheumatic complaints, can be treated externally with comfrey.

Internally it is given successfully for all kinds of respiratory tract conditions.

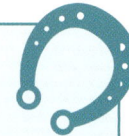

IN USE

> USED INTERNALLY

For internal use, the freshly crushed leaves are added to concentrated feed. Dried comfrey (around 30 g) can also be given with food. Symphytum has proved itself time and again in herbal remedies for all the complaints described above.

> USED EXTERNALLY

Comfrey poultices are recommended for external use. If you don't have time to prepare these yourself, you can buy them ready-made from the chemist. Comfrey ointments are also available from your vet or pharmacist.

Coneflower   *Echinacea*

The origins

The Coneflower, with its protective effects for the immune system, was already known to North American natives as a powerful remedy. They used the plant to fortify the body's defences, to combat pain, poisoning and cramps and to treat wounds.

The coneflower was brought to Europe in the 18th century. Here it was valued especially in homeopathy, where to this day it has been proving its worth. Since the mid-20th century it has also been planted in Europe, to prevent it becoming extinct in the wild.

When it grows in the garden, its beautiful flowers can be enjoyed and its roots used for medicinal purposes.

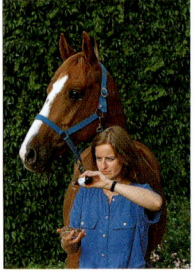

Most often, coneflower is given in the form of drops.

Medicinal properties

The best known and perhaps most important effect is the activation of the immune system. In some cases, when used at the right time, coneflower can substitute for antibiotic treatment. Many of its constituents are responsible for its powerful action: echinacin, tannins, flavonoids, resins and essential oils in combination with vitamin C strengthen the body's own defences and activate the production of blood.

In cases of obstinate infections and chronic inflammation in particular, Echinacea should be given over a lengthy period.

When used externally, it inhibits the penetration of bacteria and promotes wound healing.

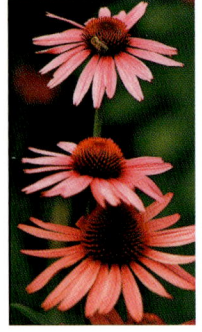

Coneflower for horses

As in humans, the pre-eminent property is strengthening the immune defences. Infections of every kind can be treated with Echinacea. You can discuss its use with your vet as an addition to any prescribed antibiotics.

Coneflower has proven itself as an excellent preventive. Whenever coughs or other infectious maladies occur in your stable, protect your horse with regular doses.

Externally it acts on infected wounds, fungal infections and especially eye and mouth inflammation.

Coneflower is used with great success to treat horses. Many vets and natural health professionals no longer want to be without it.

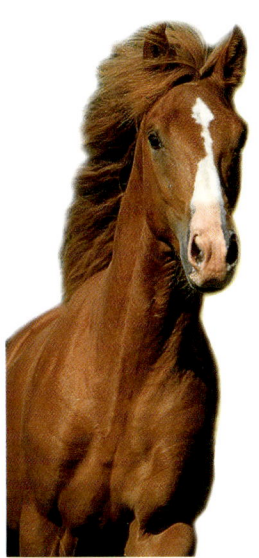

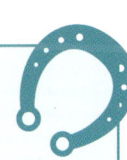

IN USE

> USED INTERNALLY

Coneflower is available these days in a wide variety of forms.

You can mix around 20 g of chopped-up roots into your horse's food every day.

As drops or juice, it can be drizzled onto dry bread or occasionally sugar and fed by hand.

The drops contain alcohol. I have a suspicion that my horses like this form more than any other.

> USED EXTERNALLY

Echinacea ointment belongs in every medicine cabinet, both at home and in the stable for external application. The diluted pressed juice is dabbed on wounds. Both the juice and the drops can be taken by the rider and the horse together.

D

Dandelion

The origins

> Effective in
laminitis
> Helps with
rheumatism
> Blood-
cleansing
> Helps with
skin and coat
problems

Taraxacum officinale

The dandelion is mentioned from the 15th century onwards. Presumably it was not recognised as a medicinal herb in antiquity. It was regarded as an incomparable remedy for wounds and its diuretic effect was described by apothecaries of that period. Today, the dandelion is very popular and occurs widely in Europe. However, it is also found in Asia and North America. The rootstock and the serrate leaves are used in natural medicine. In the spring we delight to see the pretty yellow flowers, and children love the 'blowballs' or 'clocks'. In times of hardship, roasted dandelion roots were brewed and drunk as a coffee substitute.

Medicinal properties

The dandelion is utilised in many ailments and complaints. It contains tannins, bitter substances, essential oils, provitamin A, vitamins B and C and important mineral salts. It has a proven effect as a blood-cleansing and stomach-fortifying remedy and in liver disorders, rheumatism and chronic eczema.

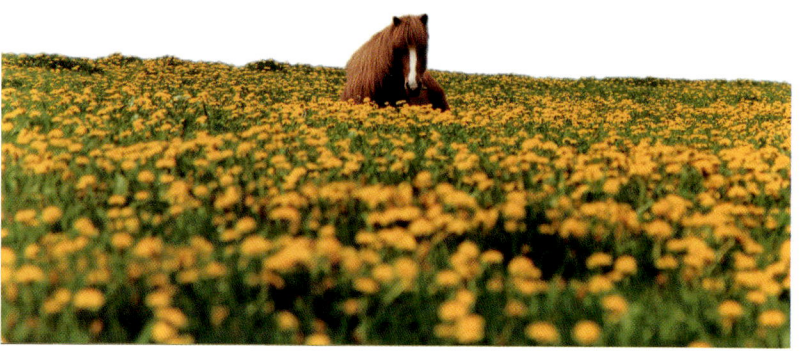

IN USE

Dandelion is best fresh from the meadow. Some horses even dig up the roots, and you can help your horse in this. Dandelion can be dried and then served as an infusion. The roots are also used, fresh or dried. Dandelion is contained in many herbal mixtures, and the infusion is available from pharmacies. As a remedy for warts, the sap of the stem has to be as fresh as possible.

> DOSAGE

Add around 30 g fresh dandelion to food or make an infusion with around 50 g dried dandelion.

> USED INTERNALLY

Mix fresh dandelion or infusion into food.

> USED EXTERNALLY

Drizzle warts with fresh dandelion sap. Dandelion sap is best given on a sterile gauze swab.

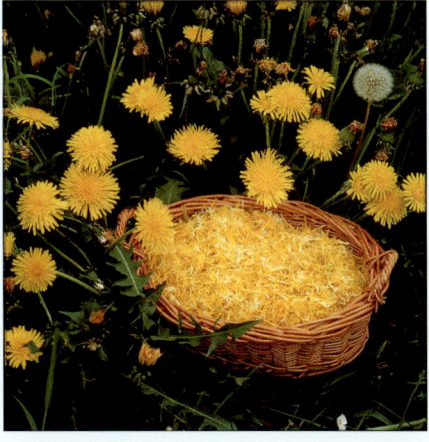

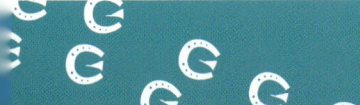

Dandelion salad is coming back into fashion and enriches our meals. A spring treatment course with dandelion is an old home remedy. It improves cholesterol levels, acts as a purgative and alleviates varicose veins and haemorrhoids.

Warts can be combated by drizzling with dandelion sap.

Dandelion for horses

Dandelion should not be absent from any horse pasture. Most horses like eating not only the leaves but also the flowers, thus treating themselves to a blood-cleansing spring cure. Dandelion has a higher vitamin A content than the popular carrot, improves the appetite and is a healthy food supplement. For rheumatic complaints, skin problems and laminitis, build dandelion into the daily menu. If your horse suffers from warts, try external treatment with dandelion sap and Thuja, which helps in almost all cases.

> Boosts the metabolism
> Good for spavin
> Significant improvement in osteoarthritis

Devil's claw   *Harpagophytum procumbens*

The origins

Devil's claw comes from hot South Africa. Its original home was the deserts of Namibia and South Africa (the Kalahari). The plant derives its name from its woody fruits, which attach themselves to objects with their hooks and disperse in this way. They are collected after the rainy season, and were used as a remedy quite early on. Traditionally, the natives regarded the devil's claw as an effective medicine for liver, gall bladder, urinary and kidney problems.

Medicinal properties

The bitter substances and flavonoids contained in the plant offer supportive therapy for joint and ligament problems.

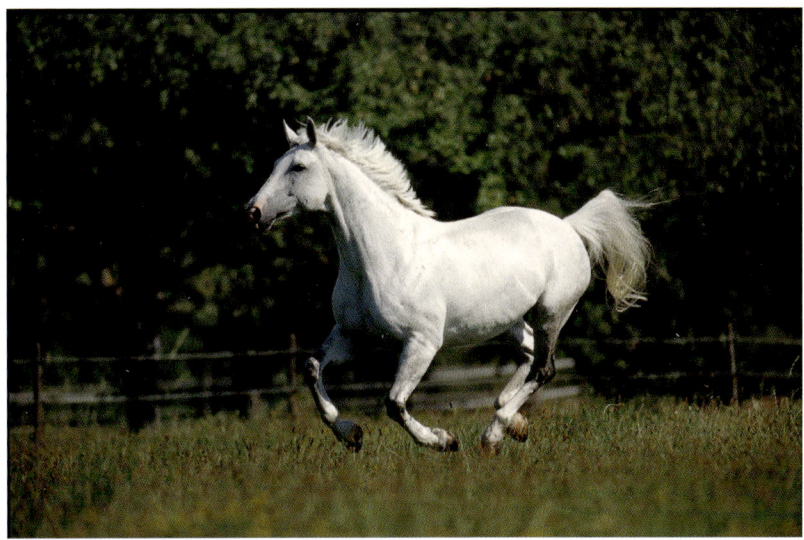

Pure joy of movement in a brisk gallop on the pasture.

Arthritis and osteoarthritis, which are associated with pain and inflammation, can be treated with devil's claw as can all other degenerative joint disorders and inflammatory bone changes. Germany is one of the main consumers of devil's claw. Investigations conducted in that country have shown that the plant's anti-inflammatory and analgesic action is comparable to that of cortisone and phenylbutazone, but without their side-effects. As the natives in Africa already knew, devil's claw is a diuretic and it boosts the liver's metabolism. In addition, it improves the appetite.

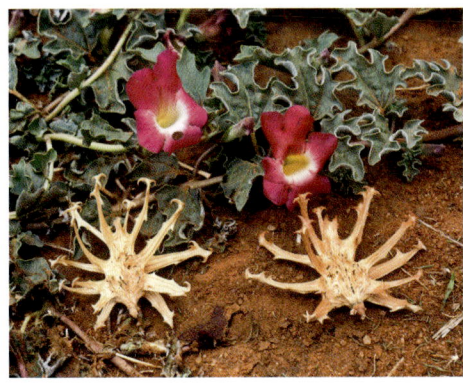

Devil's claw for horses

A comparative study in horses was conducted in France as far back as the mid-1990s. One study group suffering from spavin received a devil's claw extract, the other was given phenylbutazone. The results were amazing: the ankle-bending test, lameness while trotting and pain when turning were significantly better in the devil's claw group than in the control group treated conventionally. I carried out the test recently in three elderly horses suffering from osteoarthritis, and fed them devil's claw for some weeks. They are a 23-year-old Icelandic mare, an 18-year-old Haflinger and a 24-year-old warmblood mare. In all three horses I noticed significant improvement in symptoms and much more joy in movement.

IN USE

> USED INTERNALLY

Give horses around 15–20 grams daily. It is advisable to give the granulate over an extended period, since a visible effect comes about only after three weeks or so. Devil's claw is not a horse's favourite food, and it would be tastiest in combination with a little mash. Less picky eaters can be outsmarted with fruit vinegar, tea or honey in food.

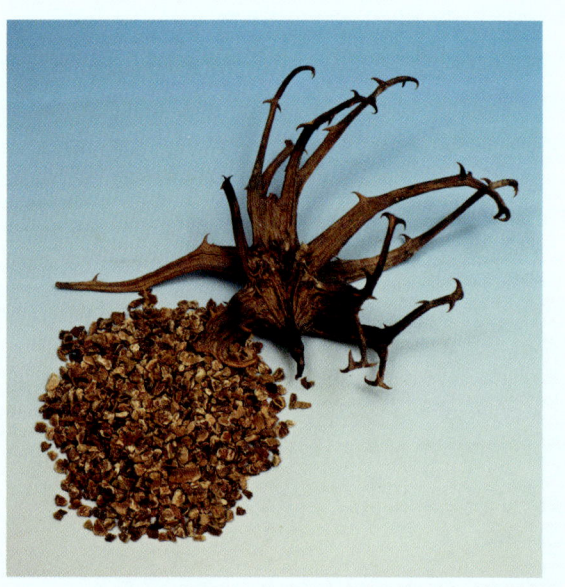

Elderberry

Sambucus nigra

Black elder

The origins

The elder was a sacred plant for the old Germanic tribes. And in the Dark Ages, the good spirits living in the trees protected people and animals from pestilence, fire and misfortune.

It is for good reason that the elder shrub or tree is praised in many old folk songs, since everything it provides is of great utility to man and beast. As greening for the home and for the stable, also as fencing for the pasture, it keeps midges and other pests away. Its flowers and fruit have manifold uses today as they have done for centuries. Before the invention of refrigerators, the elder was a reliable source of vitamins for the winter.

> Excellent vitamin source for the winter
> Helps in respiratory tract ailments

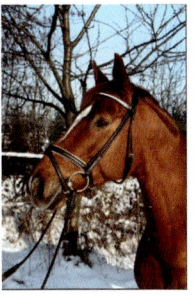

Healthy through the winter with a high vitamin supply.

Medicinal properties

The versatile blossoms provide essential oils, tannins, flavonoids and mucilage. Elderflower tea boosts the immune system and acts as a preventive against colds. Moreover, it has an attested sweat-inducing, blood-purifying and mildly laxative effect. Blossoms baked in pancake batter are healthy and tasty: a delicious recipe from Bavaria. The berries are characterised by a high content of vitamins A and C. Moreover, they contain essential oils, flavonoids, tannins and mucilage. Their antipyretic and diuretic effects are utilised especially in the form of juice. However, they can also be made into delicious wine, jam and jelly. Even the leaves are processed into oil and ointments, and help combat inflammation and haemorrhoids. Elderberry bark is a mild laxative. The shrub is a wonderful addition to the domestic garden, beautiful when planted in front of the kitchen window.

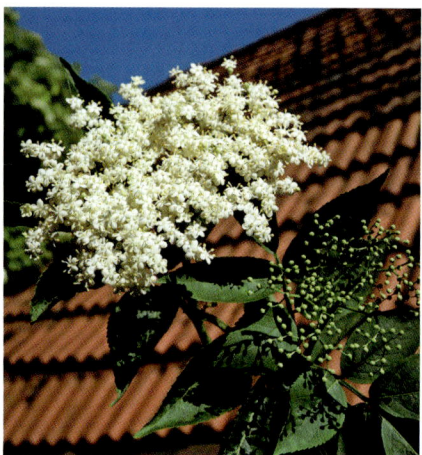
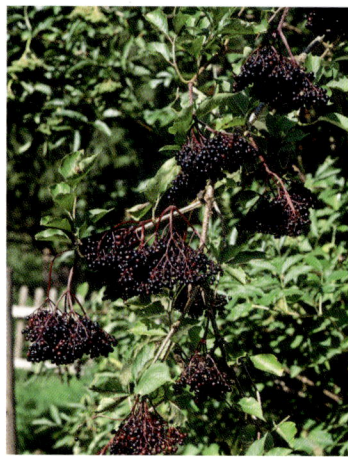

Elderberry for horses

The elder's sweat-inducing effect is, of course, undesirable in the case of horses, therefore you should not give them too much. The flowers are beneficial in disorders of the respiratory tract. Since (like the fruits) they contain valeric acid, they have a significant calming effect, including in horses. The fruit has a mild laxative and diuretic effect, and is ideal for preventing constipation colic, for example when the diet is changed in the autumn/winter from grazing to hay and straw. Do not underestimate the fruits as a good vitamin source, for horses too: the supply of vitamins A and C is not exactly abundant in winter, and this is a good preventive solution.

IN USE

> USED INTERNALLY

Provide 30–50 g of blossoms per day. Mixing with other herbs is definitely recommended. Give up to 150 g of berries per day, for example together with rosehips.

Eucalyptus

Eucalyptus globulus

> For coughs and head colds
> For brittle hooves and toe crack
> To improve the air in the stable

The origins

Eucalyptus trees can grow to 100 metres in height. Their original home is Australia, where they are greatly appreciated by the indigenous fauna. Today they also grow in southern Europe, Africa, South America and Asia. Their long roots draw up ground water, therefore eucalyptus trees have been planted widely to drain swamps.

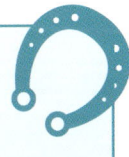

IN USE

> USED INTERNALLY

Food cough mixtures for horses always contain eucalyptus. Eucalyptus licking stones are also available nowadays. They can be recommended, but our horses eat them up in one day.

> USED EXTERNALLY

Eucalyptus in the form of pure essential oil is becoming ever more popular, especially in aromatherapy. For a sick horse, the oil can be simply placed in the stable, or sprayed with an atomiser in order to improve the air. There are inhalers for horses, but a bucket and a blanket are always to hand and are fine when nothing else is around. For inhalation, place a little hay in a bucket, drizzle a couple of drops of eucalyptus oil over it and pour boiling water on top. Then place the bucket as close as possible to the mouth and nose, and let the horse inhale until no more water vapour rises up.

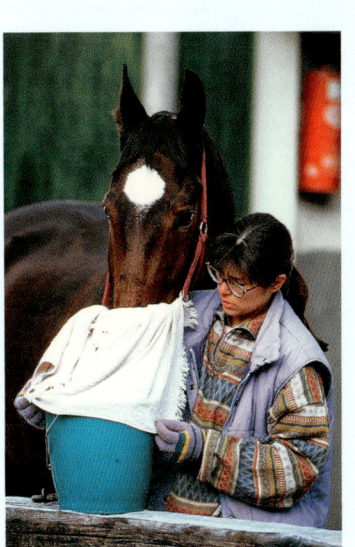

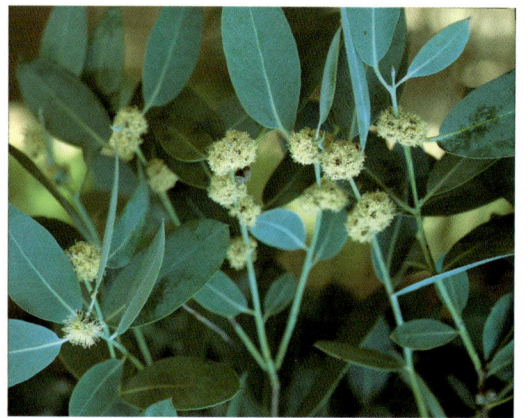

Medicinal properties

The eucalyptus tree is very popular thanks to its strong aroma and its medicinal properties. The long, sickle-shaped leaves contain essential oils. Among the known active substances, eucalyptol is the most intense. It is offered in many formats with syrup, pastilles, capsules and solutions for injection being the most common forms of administration. The tannins, essential oils and resins act in particular on the respiratory organs and the upper respiratory tract. Eucalyptus helps in cases of fever, asthma, bronchitis and frontal sinusitis. Products containing eucalyptus oil are swallowed, inhaled or used as a rub or poultice.

A TIP FROM THE VET

Vaporising a eucalyptus–water mixture improves hygiene and the air in the stable.

Eucalyptus for horses

Eucalyptus is familiar as a cough remedy. It loosens tough phlegm and has a relaxing effect. Get your coughing horse to inhale it regularly. In addition to veterinary procedures, bronchitis, asthma and head colds should always be treated with inhalations. Eucalyptus in a mild ointment base is also easy to rub into the nostrils. In case of brittle hooves and toe cracks, eucalyptus with laurel oil can be painted on the hooves.

Don't forget eucalyptus oil as protection against flies. In combination with fruit vinegar, garlic, tea tree oil and optionally lavender, one can really get to grips with the horse's adversaries.

Evening primrose

Oenothera biennis

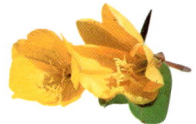

The origins

In Europe, the evening primrose has been at home only since 1612 when it was first grown in Padua's botanical garden, from where it spread to central Europe. Originally it comes from North America. The native Americans admired the evening primrose as a remedy and used it to treat the widest variety of ailments, including infections, gynaecological disorders, obesity and even snake bites.

In Europe, the evening primrose was prepared as a tasty vegetable and like black salsify was dressed with vinegar and oil.

> > Helps to combat summer eczema
> > Benefits dander and scurf
> > Good for pressure sores and minor wounds

Medicinal properties

The healing effect of evening primrose on the skin was recognised only in recent years.

The roots, stems and leaves contain tannins, flavonoids and mucilage that soothe the stomach and intestines and are used to heal wounds. The prized oil of the evening primrose, however, is contained in the seeds and has a high level of the valuable gamma-linolenic acid. It is used primarily for skin problems such as neurodermatitis, eczema, pruritus and scaly skin.

Evening primrose oil has been shown to lower cholesterol levels, cleanse the blood and act as an antispasmodic.

A TIP FROM THE VET

Evening primrose oil can be used as an alternative remedy for summer eczema.

IN USE

> USED EXTERNALLY

Evening primrose oil is applied to the clean, dry skin or coat. Horses also appreciate a short massage.

Evening primrose oil for horses

In horses, treating the skin and the coat are the most important uses of evening primrose oil.

Summer eczema, scaly skin, scurf, pruritus and sensitive areas such as the withers and areas subjected to girth pressure can be treated with the oil.

A mixture of evening primrose oil, apricot oil and Aloe vera can be made and used to treat all small or large skin injuries. Burdock root oil, too, should not be forgotten here.

Evening primrose oil is also tried and tested in horses with long leg feathering. In open stables, often the care of such long hair is rather arduous. When our horse Alma has very dirty legs, she is washed down well with an Aloe vera cleansing lotion. Once she has been towelled dry, she is massaged carefully with evening primrose oil mixture and her coat brushed smooth. In this way, horses can be prevented from rubbing the hair off their legs.

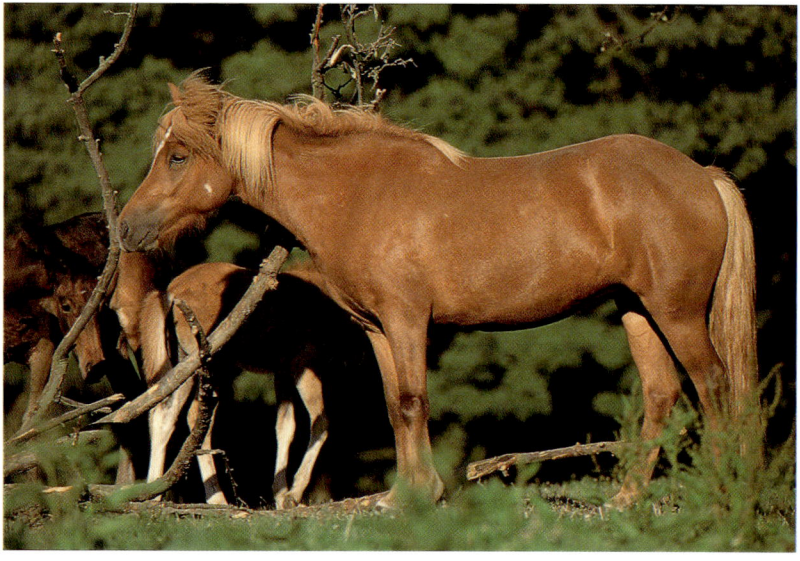

Horses suffering from eczema benefit from coat treatment with evening primrose oil.

Eyebright

Euphrasia officinalis

> Helps in eye inflammation
> Helps in disorders of the upper respiratory tract

The origins

The name Euphrasia comes from the Greek, and means joy or wellbeing. Eyebright was valued in the 12th century by St. Hildegard of Bingen. Today, it is recommended by natural healing practitioners as the most important internal and external herbal remedy for eye disorders, however you should always consult your vet.

Medicinal properties

Eyebright has an anti-inflammatory effect on all mucosal tissues. Its ingredients – iridoid glycosides, phenylpropane glycosides, flavonoids, tannins and alkaloids – have a calming and analgesic effect, especially in the eye region.

Eyebright is used in conjunctivitis and other eye inflammations and in case of a sty, itching, catarrh, mouth and throat inflammation, coughing and hoarseness. The solution used to bathe the eyes should not be made too strong. The simplest method is to use ready-made products from the pharmacy, where you can also buy eyebright tea.

A TIP FROM THE VET

If the eye is inflamed, first check to rule out a foreign body in the eye or a severe corneal injury.

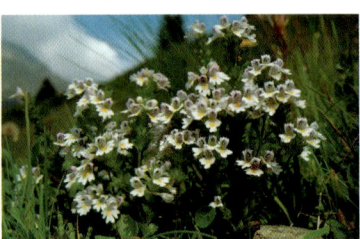

Eyebright for horses

In horses too, of course, eyebright is used primarily to treat the eyes. Horses sense the pain-relieving and calming effect at once, and mostly are well-behaved when having their eyes bathed. I always keep eyebright in the stable for immediate use in the event of an eye inflammation. Especially in the summer, when often the eyes water due to irritation by flies, daily bathing with eyebright is very helpful. Stubborn eye inflammation can be treated with eyebright internally and externally, including on top of veterinary procedures.

Disorders of the upper respiratory tract also respond very well to Euphrasia.

IN USE

Liquid eyebright preparations are available from pharmacies.

> USED EXTERNALLY

Eyebright in liquid form can be used straight or diluted. Of course, you can also make a decoction from the plant and use it instead of the commercial product.

The eyes are bathed carefully with eyebright or covered with a compress. Always use a boiled tea towel or a sterile gauze swab.

> USED INTERNALLY

For internal administration in disorders of the upper respiratory tract, it is beneficial to give the horse a tea or add 20 to 30 g dried leaves to food. Horses can be given a herbal preparation of Euphrasia, which you can buy at the pharmacy, but always consult your vet.

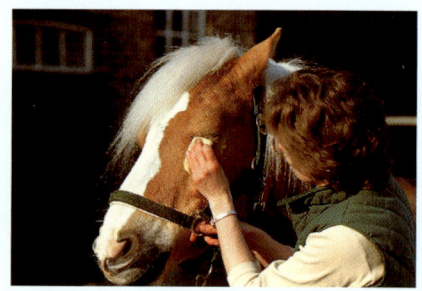

Fennel (wild)   *Foeniculum vulgare*

F

The origins

The original home of fennel is the sunny Mediterranean region. In central Europe it has established itself in the wild only in a few places. Unless you look carefully, it is easy to confuse with the related dill. The fresh leaves, roots and fruit of fennel are used as herbal remedies. The fruit contains an essential oil with good gastric and antispasmodic properties. Cooks value the strong aroma of fennel as an ideal condiment.

> *Used as an antispasmodic in gastrointestinal problems*
> *Promotes the loosening of phlegm in coughs*
> *Has wound-healing properties*

Medicinal properties

Fennel is especially well known in paediatrics. Its mild effect on the digestive system and its sweetish flavour make it a popular children's tea. In addition to essential oils, it contains vitamins A, B and C and several minerals. Among fennel's medical properties, its antispasmodic, appetite-boosting and digestion-promoting effects are particularly noteworthy. Fennel encourages milk production and is an expectorant used for coughs and bronchitis. Its wound-healing effect is valued in the treatment of abscesses and eye injuries.

TIP FOR THE RIDER

Naturally, fennel tea helps the rider too with gastric problems and coughs, and should be present in every home.

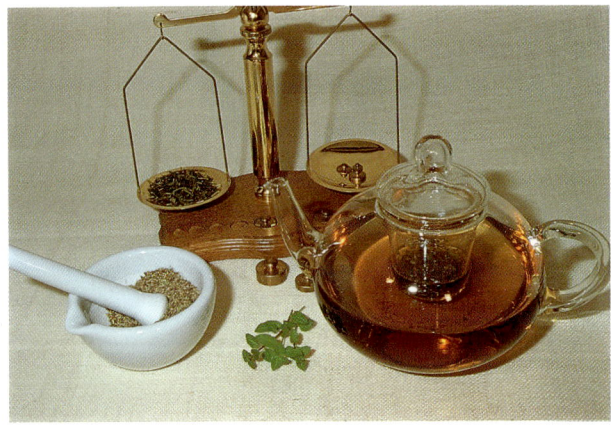

Antispasmodic fennel tea is drunk willingly not only by children but also by horses.

Fennel for horses

A mixture of anise, fennel and caraway is optimal as a digestive tea. Moreover, all horses accept its flavour. In any form of flatulence caused by a change of

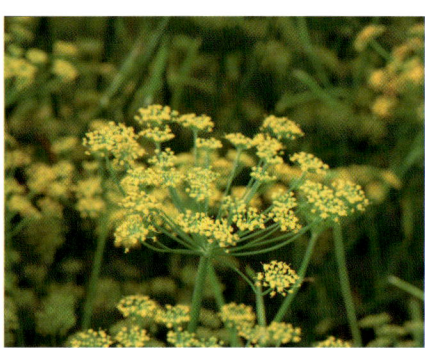

food at the start of the grazing season, fennel soothes the gastrointestinal tract thanks to its antispasmodic properties. All respiratory ailments benefit from fennel. Utilise its expectorant effect to deal with coughs, bronchitis and rhinorrhoea. Externally, you can bathe wounds and abscesses with fennel tea. Especially for eye problems in combination with eyebright, fennel offers quick help. Mares with foals are often given fennel to encourage milk production, and the antispasmodic ingredients are also useful for the foal.

IN USE

> USED INTERNALLY

I prefer to give fennel as a tea or a tea mixture together with anise and caraway. Horses are happy to drink it, and its essential oils develop their effect optimally thanks to the hot water. Fennel is added to nearly all herbal mixtures for horses.

> USED EXTERNALLY

For external use and for inhalation, prepare a stronger tea and let it cool down.

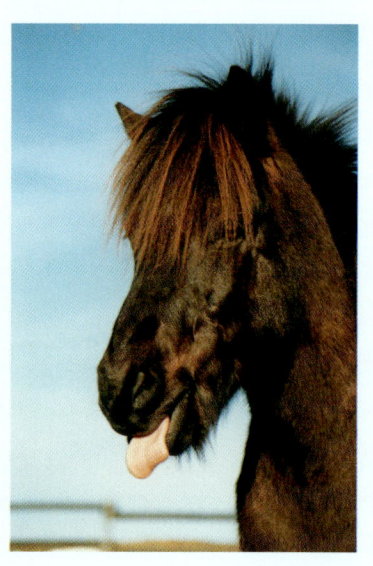

Fenugreek

Greek hay

Trigonella foenum graecum

The origins

Fenugreek has been cultivated since antiquity in southwest Asia and the eastern Mediterranean region. It was introduced to central Europe in the 9th century and also planted there. The seeds, which have a high mucilage content, are used in medicine and in naturopathy. Due to environmental pollution, fenugreek is only rarely found growing in the wild. As a cultivated plant, it occurs worldwide. As the name Greek hay suggests, it is also commonly used as animal feed.

Medicinal properties

The dried seeds contain mucilage, saponins, bitter substances and essential oils. Fenugreek oil increases the appetite and promotes the uptake of fat. Therefore it is often given after an illness to achieve weight gain. It is an excellent remedy in diabetes, since it lowers blood sugar levels. Externally, fenugreek is beneficial for boils and nail inflammations. In breastfeeding mothers, it is recommended to boost milk production.

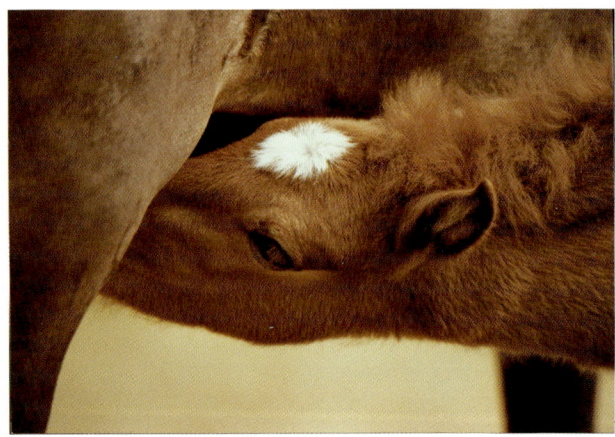

Fenugreek for horses

In other parts of the world, fenugreek is a sought-after food plant. Here we can use only the seeds for our horses. If you have a thin horse who despite

The seeds of fenugreek encourage milk production.

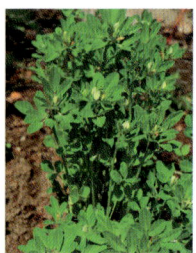

all your care has a dull coat and also suffers from poor hooves, try fenugreek. The plant's chemistry has some similarity with cod liver oil, and the same goes for its effect. Horses put on weight, gain a beautiful shiny coat and healthy, solid hooves. Their general condition improves and the immune system is boosted. In lactating mares, the milk flow is stimulated. Don't give fenugreek to pregnant mares. Respiratory tract disorders are positively influenced in combination with garlic and other herbs.

IN USE

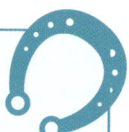

Fenugreek is available nowadays in feed and herbal mixtures for horses, and thus is easy to use. The seeds can be purchased commercially and added to the horse's food (up to 100 g per day). If you have a large garden or room in the pasture, you can also plant fenugreek yourself.

> USED INTERNALLY

Add fenugreek seeds to food.

> USED EXTERNALLY

For rheumatic complaints, it is a good idea to make poultices with the crushed seeds.

> DOSAGE

Up to around 100 g fenugreek seeds per day.

Field horsetail

Scouring rush

Equisetum arvense

> Important for a robust immune system
> Helps in congestion and oedema
> Long-term treatment for coat and hooves

The origins

The horsetails are one of the oldest plant families. Fossilised specimens have been found that are older than 300 million years.

Even in antiquity, field horsetail was used as a medicinal product for dehydration and to stop bleeding. Later, the German priest and naturopath Sebastian Kneipp adopted this approach and used the horsetail plant for 'blood cleansing' in his cures. The name 'scouring rush' reminds us that the green shoots growing in summer can be used to polish metal. Farmers do not like the horsetail, regarding it as a weed. The roots of the plant reach extremely deep into the soil and are difficult to get rid of. From June to August, the green parts above ground may be used for making tea.

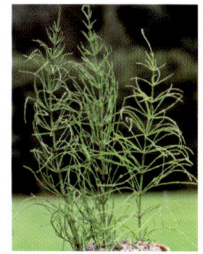

Medicinal properties

The best known ingredient of horsetail is silicic acid (silicon dioxide in water). Its effect on connective tissue, on the elasticity of the skin and on the make-up of bones, teeth and nails makes it indispensable not only in natural medicine but also in natural cosmetics. Potassium, alkaloids, saponins and flavonoids are other valuable substances in this plant. This versatile 'weed' stimulates the body both internally and externally. As a gentle diuretic, horsetail can help with kidney and bladder problems. It is useful for boosting the immune system, and it supports treatments for asthma, skin inflammations, rheumatism, circulation disorders and frostbite. Externally, it is used as a poultice or a bath additive, for example to help with skin problems.

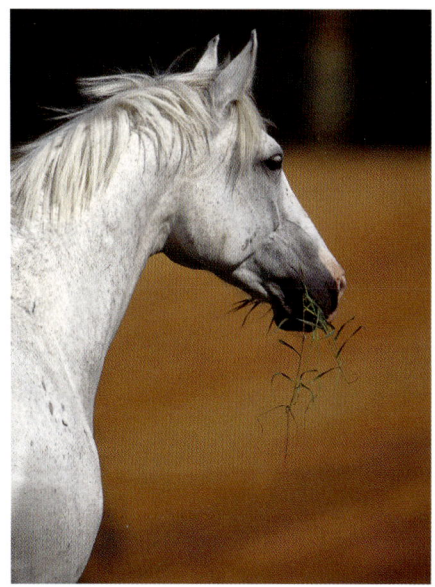

Horsetail contributes to a healthy coat.

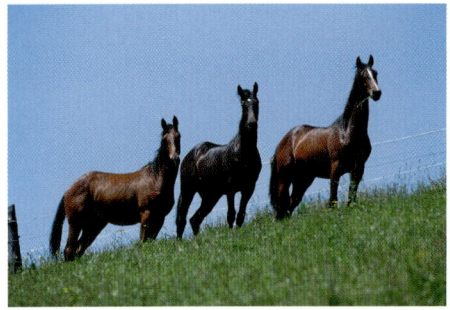

Enjoying the pasture without eczema.

Horsetail for horses

For horses too, horsetail is recommended for kidney inflammation and its mild dehydrating effect helps with congestion.

Its positive effect on the coat and hooves can be utilised if the horse suffers from eczema, poorly growing hooves or other skin problems. In cases of summer eczema, you should start using it a few weeks before the grazing season. Coat and hoof problems always require long-term therapy.

IN USE

> USED EXTERNALLY

In horses too, a decoction can offer relief from several skin problems.

> USED INTERNALLY

25–50 g is given internally per day. Unless you are very familiar with the plant in nature, you need to obtain it commercially. It has a poisonous relative, the marsh horsetail, and confusing the two plants would be fatal.

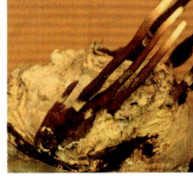

Fungi

The origins

Traditional Chinese medicine (TCM) has been working with medicinal mushrooms for thousands of years. Fungi, including mushrooms, are a very special group of living organisms: they are biologically unusual, belonging neither to the plant nor the animal kingdom. In Asia, medicinal mushrooms are used to prevent and treat severe illnesses. Some fungi were regarded as particularly valuable since they were rare and difficult to find, for example reishi, the emperor's mushroom. Reishi was weighed out with gold and was intended only for rulers. For some years now, it has been possible to cultivate mushrooms such as reishi on a larger scale, so that today it is available to all sectors of the population.

> *Intensive stimulation for the immune system*
> *Have a balancing effect on the nervous system*

Medicinal properties

Medicinal mushrooms contain a wide range of highly efficacious ingredients with high bioavailability. These mushrooms regulate disharmonies in the body, which are the reason for many illnesses, in a unique way. Medicinal mushrooms are ideally suited both for prevention and for treatment in certain acute conditions (usually without side-effects). Reishi is especially rich in vitamins, minerals, trace elements and amino acids. It has an incredibly positive effect on allergies. Moreover, it is known as an absolute anti-aging star. Medicinal mushrooms stimulate the immune system intensively. Their action is detoxifying, antibacterial and antiviral. After taking any necessary strong medications, they stabilise internal organs such as the liver and kidneys. Valuable polysaccharides (sugar molecules), vitamins, minerals and trace elements restore the body's equilibrium.

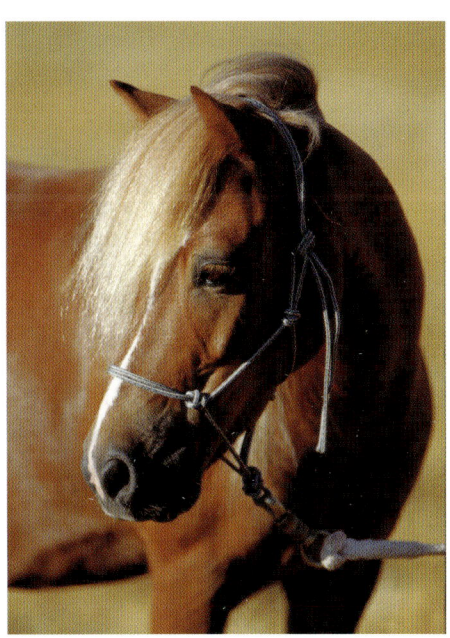

Fully alert and motivated.

Medicinal mushrooms for horses

Vets and natural health professionals have also been interested in medicinal mushrooms for some years now. In particular, reishi (or lingzhi, which means 'divine mushroom of immortality') and Cordyceps (caterpillar fungus)

CAUTION

Important for tournament horses: Cordyceps is on the doping list!

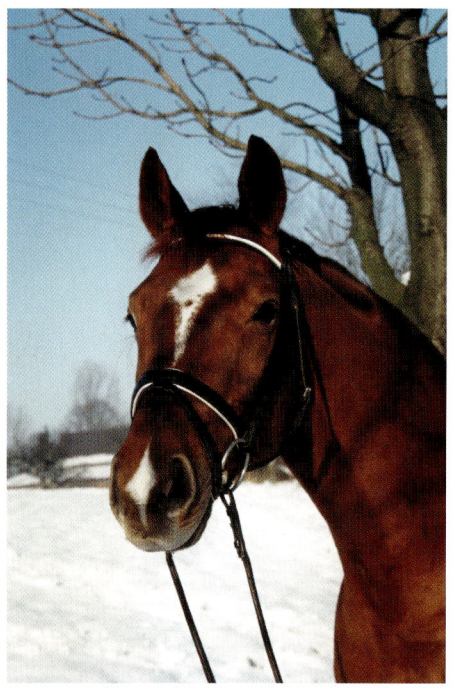

Cordyceps is a wonderful fortifying tonic for horses.

have made a name for themselves in the treatment of horses, dogs, cats and other animals. Their tremendous fortifying effect on the immune system is always emphasised. There are, after all, many ailments that are associated with a weak immune system. In particular, abnormal equine behaviour can be treated with medicinal mushrooms. Anxiety, aggression, shock and neurasthenia have a variety of causes, and it is not always easy to determine the decisive one in any given case. Trying reishi, for example, could well be worthwhile. It promotes inner peace and the equilibrium of the nervous system. Nowadays, allergies in horses are very often a problem. Here too, lingzhi can be used successfully. Old horses, like people, suffer from a variety of minor ailments. Reishi is certainly a fountain of youth. Aging processes are delayed, coat problems and disorders of the musculoskeletal system remedied. In Japan, reishi is approved as a medication against cancer. Sadly, there isn't enough space here to list all the options that mushroom therapy offers. Cordyceps is regarded as a special fortifying tonic. In horses it enhances performance, detoxifies and is beneficial in lung and kidney diseases. Bacterial infections and rheumatism too, respond to it well.

IN USE

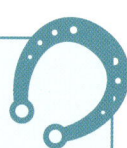

> USED INTERNALLY

Medicinal mushrooms can be prepared in two ways: powder and extract.

The powder consists of dried and ground mushrooms. All the biological substances, vitamins and minerals are retained. Extracts are more expensive than pure mushroom powder, since their concentration is 30 to 50 times higher. Both forms are available commercially.

Garlic   *Allium sativum*

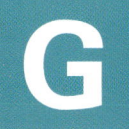

The origins

Garlic hung over the door and the window repels vampires, witches and demons. Even if we no longer believe this, garlic should not be absent from any stable. It is one of the oldest medicinal plants, and its origins can be traced back over 5,000 years. The Romans, the Greeks and the old Germanic peoples used garlic as a spice and a remedy. Nations that eat a lot of garlic are healthier and live longer.

Having arrived from the Orient, it is now also grown in on all continents.

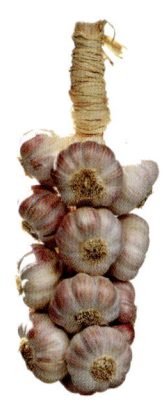

Medicinal properties

Many different active ingredients have been found in garlic. These include amino acids, enzymes, allicin and hormone-like substances.

It is the bactericidal action in particular that makes garlic such a useful remedy. It kills off pathogenic bacteria and fungi in the gut and in this way prevents fermentation processes. In addition, garlic dilates the blood vessels and improves the circulatory properties of the blood. Furthermore, it has a relaxing effect on cramp-like pain. Garlic is reputed to inhibit the growth of tumours and to flush poisons from the body. Externally, garlic can be utilised to disinfect minor wounds, fight fungi and alleviate insect bites.

> To improve general well-being
> Protects against insects and severe worm infestation
> Restores intestinal equilibrium following a course of antibiotics

Suckling mares
should be given
garlic only in small
quantities. The
milk must not take
on the flavour,
otherwise the
foal may become
confused and even
reject the milk.

Garlic for horses

Even avowed opponents of herbal remedies have, at one time or another, used garlic when looking after their horses. Nowadays it is contained in many food mixtures, herbal teas and natural insect repellents. Garlic should be fed over a prolonged period, then it can unfold its full effect since the aroma that people are not so fond of is also unpopular with flies and midges. And that's precisely what benefits our horses. The sulphur flowing out through the skin and the mouth keeps those annoying pests away.

Moreover, garlic prevents ailments of the respiratory tract, ensures the balance of intestinal flora and protects against severe worm infestations. If antibiotic treatment is required, it can be followed by giving garlic to restore the balance of the intestines and of all other organs.

You will notice in your horses a marked improvement in general well-being. Their activity and concentration will increase, whereas their nervousness, anxiety and sensitivity will decrease.

IN USE

> USED INTERNALLY

A fresh clove is the most effective. It is chopped up fine and mixed into food. A little fruit vinegar or tea can hide the initially unusual taste. Naturally, you can also give ready-to-use powder or a herbal mixture containing garlic. The only important thing is to use garlic over a prolonged period and increase the dose as necessary.

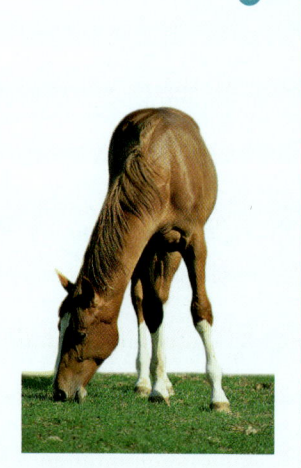

> USED EXTERNALLY

Externally, one can apply garlic as a juice or a freshly sliced clove to fungal infections, small wounds and insect bites. Garlic is also a proven remedy against ticks and lice.

Ginger

Zingiber officinale

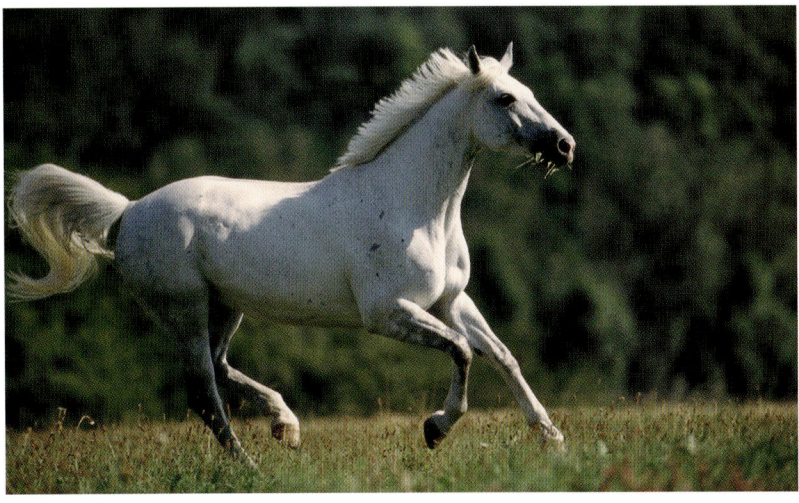

The origins

This very well-known rhizome of the ginger shrub is not only a popular spice, but is moving increasingly into the limelight as a medicinal plant. It has been known for thousands of years in Africa, and all over Asia and has been ascribed a healing action. Its unusual sharpness adds a special character to many dishes, and furthermore each one becomes significantly healthier. Ginger is said to contain more than 500 biological substances, and they can unfold their healing and constitution-improving effects in both people and animals. It is added even to sweets, although for many people, especially children, chocolate with ginger is rather an acquired taste.

> Holds intestinal bacteria and worms in check
> Good against osteoarthritis
> Ideal when mixed with devil's claw

Medicinal properties

There is an unbelievable wealth of ingredients in this unusual tuber. In addition to spicy substances known as gingerols, various essential oils

Full of vitality once again, thanks to ginger.

and resin acids, ginger contains vitamin C, zinc, magnesium, iron, calcium and potassium. Gingerols are supposed to exhibit the same action as some anti-inflammatory and analgesic medicines, for example aspirin and Equipalazone. Even in small quantities as a culinary spice, ginger is reputed to have an effect on the liver and all digestive organs. Metabolism is boosted and allergic conditions affected positively. As an alternative medicine it also helps in rheumatism, muscle pain and colds.

Ginger for horses

The list of applications in the treatment of animals reads like a miracle drug. Ginger has been used for some years now as a remedy when feeding horses. Pain, inflammation and osteoarthritis can be alleviated significantly. According to current scientific knowledge, osteoarthritis is incurable. However, its symptoms from lameness through pain can be alleviated and in part even arrested. Good results have been achieved with ginger in cases involving spavin, ringbone, laminitis, navicular syndrome and all other joint problems. Recent research even attributes improvements in equine tumours to ginger. It is always worthwhile trying to supplement and support the vet's treatment with natural remedies. Ginger can be a useful addition even in the treatment of worms. Whether it's really possible to reduce chemical deworming is something that should be checked with a stool sample in each particular case.

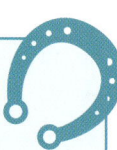

IN USE

> DOSAGE

There are as yet no reliable scientific studies about the exact dosage in horses. Experts, however, recommend a daily administration of 3 g ginger per 100 kg. In many complaints, this dose has resulted in significant improvement in symptoms.

Since ginger, like devil's claw, is not on the list of foods popular with horses and ponies, it is advisable to start slowly, get the animal used to the taste and then increase the amount. Ginger is available in granules or as a powder, although it seems to be more readily accepted as granules. The usual tricks can be resorted to: mash, carrots and apples, fruit vinegar, hay pellets and so on. Liquid ginger with additional herbs has recently become commercially available. A mixture of devil's claw and ginger is of proven benefit for osteoarthritis: do give it a try. There are some who warn against excessive doses and long-term use.

Sensitive animals may suffer from irritation of the gastric mucosa. In such cases it is important to use ginger in a controlled manner and of course keep an eye on the horse.

Ginkgo biloba

Maidenhair tree

Ginkgo biloba

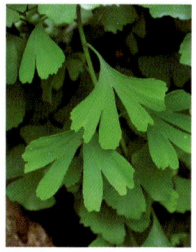

The origins

The maidenhair tree is a relict from the past. Numerous ginkgo species were common worldwide 200 million years ago. Only Ginkgo biloba remains, having survived nearly unchanged in one part of East Asia. This huge tree can grow up to 40 metres tall, and is at home today in East Asia, North America and Europe. In traditional Chinese medicine, ginkgo has long been an established remedy. But in Europe too, its leaves were used to heal wounds in earlier times. In China, the seeds are used raw or cooked for a wide range of ailments. In Europe, mainly the leaves are used in naturopathy. You can grow a ginkgo tree in your own garden – but remember those 40 metres!

> Helps to treat laminitis
> Boosts concentration
> Boosts blood circulation in the organs and limbs

Medicinal properties

The effects of ginkgo leaves derive from their main active ingredients, namely ginkgolides, bilobalides and flavonoids. The extract promotes blood circulation in the brain and in the entire body, especially in the legs. The viscosity of the blood is decreased and its oxygen uptake is increased. Depressive moods, poor concentration and deteriorating memory are improved by ginkgo. In the treatment of Alzheimer's disease, unequivocal success has been achieved with ginkgo. Headaches and dizziness caused by circulation disorders respond positively to treatment with ginkgo.

Ginkgo biloba for horses

We can utilise the circulation-promoting effect in our horses, too. Increasing the oxygen uptake improves the supply to all the organs. Horses who have difficulty concentrating during work and allow themselves to be constantly distracted, can be treated with ginkgo. Significantly better blood circulation in the extremities has been demonstrated in horses, as has an effect in shocks of all kinds. Positive experiences have been seen with laminitis.

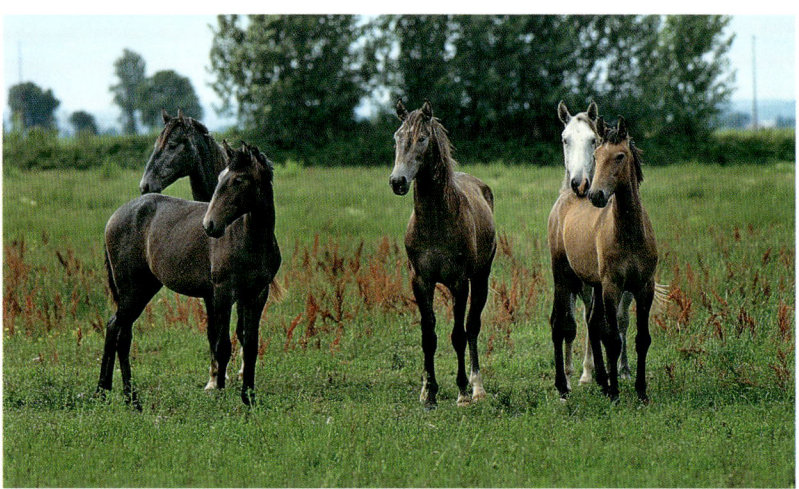

Healthy and alert horses – Ginkgo biloba helps!

IN USE

> USED INTERNALLY

It is straightforward to prepare ginkgo leaf tea. There are no side-effects and it tastes spicy and delicious. For a more intensive effect, however, the extract has to be used. You cannot produce it yourself, but you can buy it in the form of drops or tablets at the pharmacy. Your vet or alternative practitioner will have Ginkgo biloba solution for injection. Homeopathic administration to horses is recommended by natural healing practitioners, but always consult your vet.

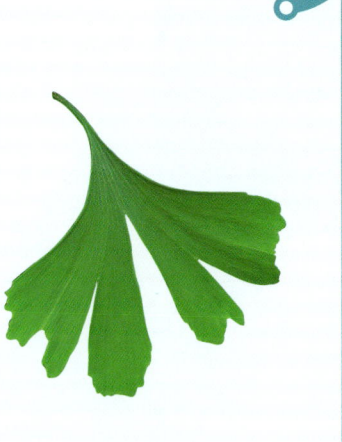

Ginseng   *Panax schinseng*

The origins

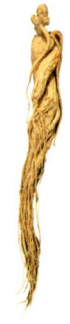

The royal medicinal plant of the Chinese emperor grew originally in the shady mountain forests of East Asia, from northern Korea and Manchuria to Nepal. Today, the plant is largely extinct in the wild, and grows almost only as a cultivated crop for medicinal purposes in Korea, China, Japan and Ukraine. Since growing ginseng is very difficult, this 'wonder root' is not exactly one of the most inexpensive natural remedies. However, a plethora of studies in the East and the West, in humans and animals, demonstrate unambiguously the healing and regenerating power of the ginseng root, and its use in many ailments is nevertheless worthwhile.

> Improves concentration and motivation
> Reduces stress
> Increases fertility
> Regulates blood pressure and metabolism

TIP FOR THE RIDER

Not only for your horse but also for yourself: if you have to meet demanding challenges or ongoing stress, treat yourself to the benefits of ginseng.

Medicinal properties

The many valuable ingredients, including essential oils, starch, sugar, pectin, biotin, vitamins B1, B2 and B12, ginsenin, panaxic acid, phosphates, trace elements and ginsenosides, make ginseng a wonder drug.

Investigations around the world have confirmed its efficacy. Ginseng affects the entire organism positively, it stimulates the central nervous system and increases the supply of oxygen. Stress is alleviated and performance boosted for a long time. Under the effect of ginseng, concentration and responsiveness are boosted and thus intellectual potential increased. Improving vitality at an advanced age, regulating blood pressure and promoting metabolism are further benefits of this small root.

IN USE

> USED INTERNALLY

Ready-to-use ginseng products for horses are available commercially. They are certainly good, but not very cheap. Ginseng is subject to strict quality control, but even so there are great price differences. Extracts are highly soluble and are offered as powder or granules. The older the root, the better the quality. Six-year-old plants are the most efficacious. Ginseng can be given with food.

The root has a distinct aroma and tastes sweet and slightly bitter at the same time. Ginseng should be taken over an extended period of time. It has no side-effects.

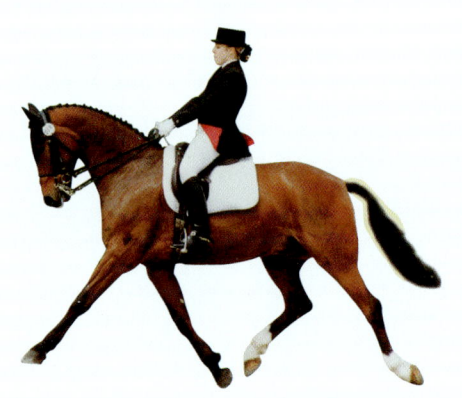

> DOSAGE

Add ginseng powder, granules or root to food according to the dosage instructions.

Ginseng for horses

Ginseng root is well-established in veterinary medicine. Give your sport horses (tournaments, training, trail rides) ginseng regularly and you will hardly recognise them. Ginseng does a good job in dealing with exhaustion, especially after an illness.

Horses undergoing endurance training can benefit greatly from ginseng. When starting young horses under saddle, this makes great demands on their concentration. They are more cooperative when taking the root extract.

Constant stress always makes ginseng treatment necessary. Siberian ginseng is preferred for increasing fertility, and is used successfully in both mares and stallions.

Think about your old horses, too. With ginseng they will remain healthy, fit and full of joy.

Goosegrass   *Galium oparine*

The origins

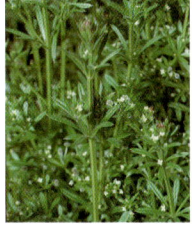

Goosegrass is much better than its reputation. It was described by the ancient Greeks as a useful plant. This rampant climber occurs all across Europe. It grows in fields, thickets and woods and climbs up fences. Its leaves and stems are used for medicinal purposes.

> *> Good for swollen legs*
> *> Beneficial in laminitis*
> *> Stops bleeding from small wounds*

Medicinal properties

Goosegrass has a positive effect on blood circulation and the lymphatic system. It contains a great deal of silica, and therefore strengthens the skin and hair. It is used, among others, for skin ulcers, jaundice and oedema. The fresh juice of the plant or a poultice of crushed leaves have haemostatic properties. It is also used to treat wounds and abscesses.

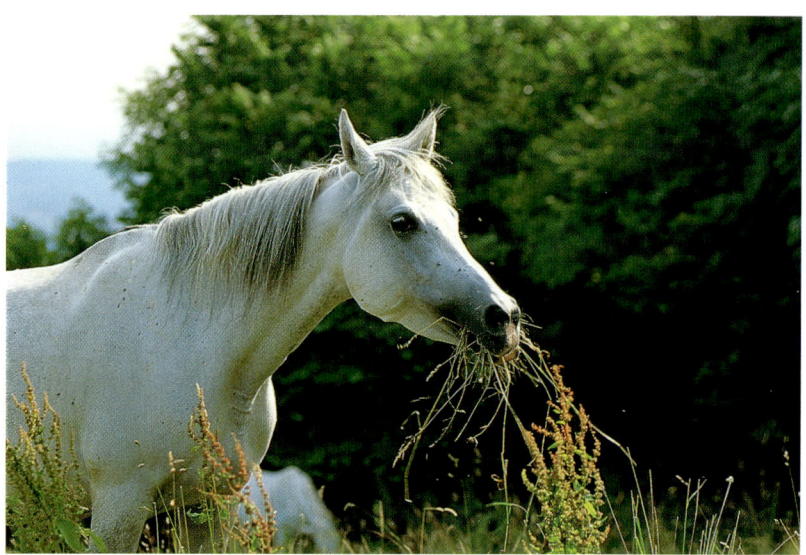

Horses eat goosegrass readily.

Goosegrass for horses

A TIP FROM THE VET

Swollen legs can have various causes, including in the region of the tendons and joints. These need to be investigated using x-rays and ultrasound.

Goosegrass is not popular with farmers and gardeners, but if you find it in a corner of the pasture, leave it be. It is good for horses, and you will find that on some days they prefer to eat it. When kept properly, horses often know what's good for them and take the nutrients made available to them of their own accord. Obviously, this doesn't apply in the stable in front of the open feed box.

In particular, if your horses have swollen legs or oedema then mow a little goosegrass and give it to them to eat. Ponies and horses suffering from laminitis should also eat goosegrass. The silica it contains is especially important for the coat and hooves. Externally, the crushed leaves can serve as first aid for small wounds.

IN USE

Goosegrass really is found all over the place, even in the city on old plots of land and along fences. There is plenty of it, and you are allowed to pick it anywhere. Farmers will be delighted if you free their field from goosegrass. You can even dry it for the winter.

> DOSAGE

Every horse can manage three handfuls of fresh goosegrass per day. As always, give around 30 g of the dried plant. On the pasture your horses know themselves how much they want.

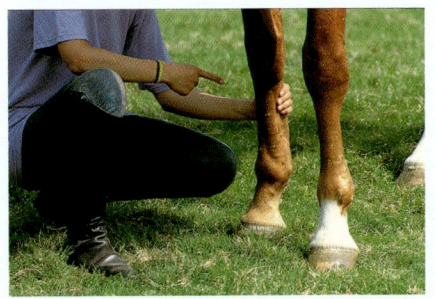

Grapefruit seed extract

Citrus paradisi

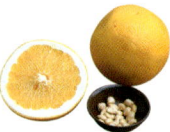

The origins

The grapefruit originated in the islands of the West Indies, according to some researchers as a cross between the pomelo and the orange. It was first identified in 1750 in Barbados.

The botanical name – literally 'citrus of paradise' – hints at the wonderful content of this plant. Until recently, the grapefruit was familiar only as a delicious source of vitamins. Now, however, further extraordinary active ingredients are being investigated.

Nowadays, grapefruit seed extract is taken for a large number of complaints and ailments. Numerous studies have confirmed the extract's broad antimicrobial effect. This is why it has entered into use as a highly effective natural remedy.

> Effectively supports deworming products
> Activates the immune system
> Helps in fungal infections and insect bites

Medicinal properties

Vitamin C is one of the most important active substances in grapefruit. It encourages cell metabolism, promotes the production of blood and boosts the body's immune system, especially important in preventing infections. Various laboratory investigations in several countries have focused in particular on grapefruit seeds, showing a growth-inhibiting effect on bacteria, viruses and fungi.

Grapefruit seed extract is used for gastrointestinal problems, fungal infection, colds and tooth and gum inflammation.

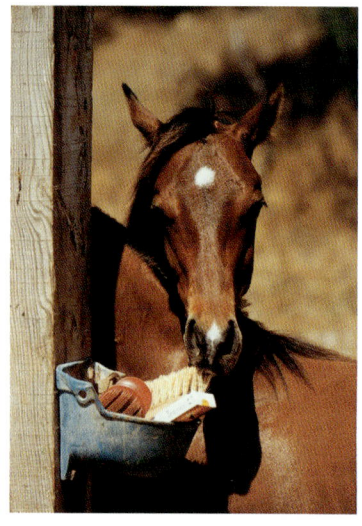

Grapefruit seed extract for horses

Grapefruit seed extract is a natural and effective way to assist conventional deworming products.

It can be used internally to treat fungal disorders. For external fungal infections, rub a few drops every day on the affected site, and bathe large areas. Smaller injuries and wounds can also be treated with grapefruit seed extract.

Spraying grapefruit seed extract on the coat repels annoying pests in the summer. If, despite this, there are insect bites of any kind at all, the extract can be rubbed in. In the summer you can spray a mixture of water and grapefruit seed extract in the stable; the odour will drive midges and flies away.

IN USE

Grapefruit seed extract in powder or liquid form is available from the pharmacy.

> USED INTERNALLY

Mix powdered or liquid extract into food.

> USED EXTERNALLY

The extract can be used externally either straight or diluted with water, as applicable in each case.

> DOSAGE

For internal use, remember the following as a rule of thumb: 0.02 ml liquid extract or 2.5 mg powder per kg of body weight. In other words, give an average-size warmblood (600 kg) 12 ml liquid extract or 1.5 g powder.

Green tea   *Thea sinensis/Camellia sinensis*

Vitality from Asia

The origins

Green tea has been a greatly valued natural remedy in Asia for thousands of years. It was first mentioned 4,700 years ago and was brought from China to Japan by Buddhist monks in the 11th century. The tea bush was originally planted in Chinese monastery gardens for medicinal purposes only. In contrast to black tea, the active ingredients in green tea are not destroyed. All the important substances, the aroma and the green colour are preserved. According to the latest scientific studies, 130 different active substances are responsible for the positive properties of green tea, including, for example, vitamins A, B, C and E, amino acids, proteins, fruit acids and trace elements such as calcium and magnesium.

Today, green tea extract is one of the most interesting complexes of active substances in naturopathy.

> *Boosts the immune system*
> *For recovering after an illness*
> *Makes up mineral losses*
> *Against summer eczema*

Medicinal properties

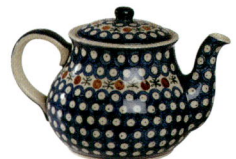

In Chinese tradition, green tea is the source of many healing, strengthening and preventive effects. Green tea preserves youth and inspires the body and the mind. According to the latest research, green tea helps slow down the ageing process 20 times more than the well-known vitamin E.

It is valued as a mental stimulant, improves concentration and boosts endurance. In addition to its internal effect, green tea also activates externally all the natural functions of the skin. It is recommended in particular for dry, irritated and allergic skin.

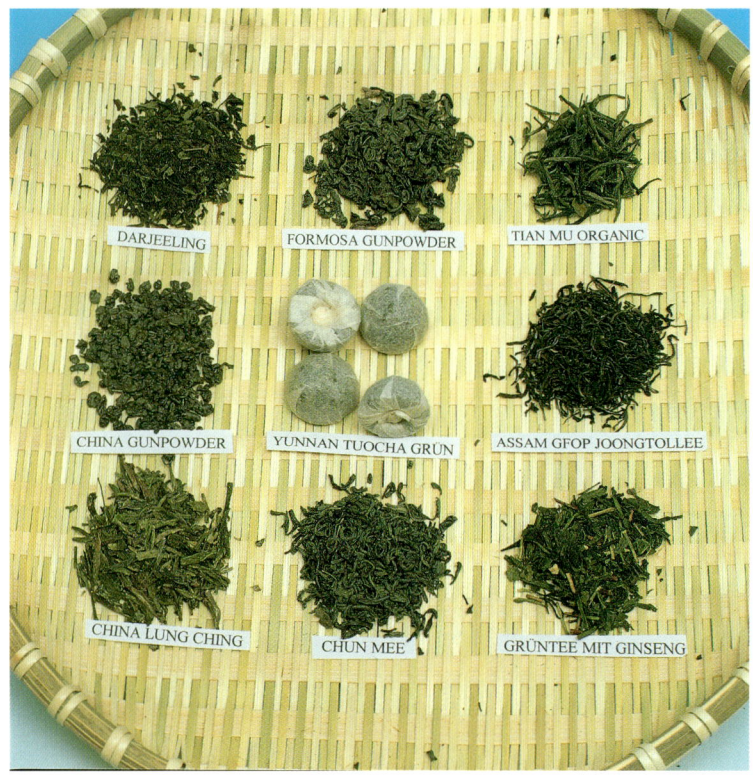

DARJEELING   FORMOSA GUNPOWDER   TIAN MU ORGANIC

CHINA GUNPOWDER   YUNNAN TUOCHA GRÜN   ASSAM GFOP JOONGTOLLEE

CHINA LUNG CHING   CHUN MEE   GRÜNTEE MIT GINSENG

Green tea for horses

As with people, green tea can be used in horses in manifold ways for internal and external treatment. Older and weak horses especially, should be given green tea every day over a prolonged period. For horses who need to recover after an illness too, a daily ration of green tea is a good tonic. The bitter substances in it stimulate the appetite and digestion, can stop diarrhoea and make up the loss of minerals. Horses under performance stress need green tea in order to improve their concentration and endurance and avoid exhaustion.

Externally, green tea is excellent for washes of all kinds, for example to treat eczema, such as summer eczema, or dry and scaly skin.

Furthermore, it can be used as a shampoo additive for the mane and tail, and in the summer to refresh the entire body.

IN USE

Add the tea to drinking water or to concentrated food.

> USED INTERNALLY

Allow two bags to steep for around five to six minutes in 0.25 to 0.5 l water.

> USED EXTERNALLY

Steep double the amount for around 10 to 15 minutes.

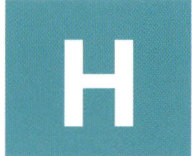

H

Hawthorn

Crataegus

The origins

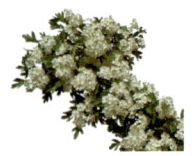

> Strengthens
the heart
> Stabilises
the circulation
> Beneficial in
laminitis

However enchanting the beauty of the hawthorn's white blossoms, it emits a very unpleasant smell which attracts flies and beetles for pollination. Hawthorn, also known as whitethorn, occurs frequently as a shrub or tree in Europe and the USA. It can reach an age of 500 to 600 years. In earlier years, the fruits were eaten during times of food shortage or used as animal fodder. The hawthorn has been used medicinally in China for more than 1,000 years. It is one of the best-known medicinal plants and is scientifically recognised.

According to superstition, hawthorn twigs above the door keep the house and stable free from disease.

Medicinal properties

Few natural remedies are as undisputed in medicine as the hawthorn, especially in the treatment of heart conditions.

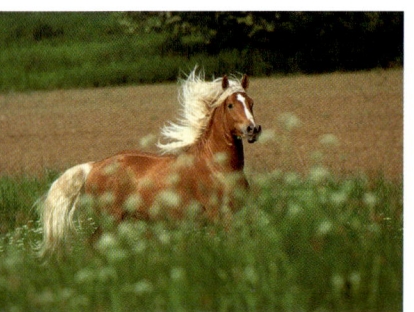

Hawthorn is also good for prevention.

The blossoms, fruits, bark and twigs contain valuable substances such as flavonoids, amines, histamine, tannins and vitamin C. The possible applications of the hawthorn are many, with the main focus on its heart-fortifying effect. Its medical properties are valued for internal and external use: it is an astringent, an antihypertensive, a febrifuge, a diuretic, and an antispasmodic, and it strengthens the blood circulation.

The hawthorn's calming effect on anxiety, nervousness, cramps and insomnia is utilised by many people.

Hawthorn for horses

If you give hawthorn to your horses, it's best to do this as long-term therapy since it needs four to six weeks to develop its effect fully. In horses too, the heart's efficiency decreases over the years. Hawthorn is outstanding in preventing and treating mild cardiac weakness. It has a positive effect on the circulation, and stabilises blood pressure.

When observing elderly horses on the pasture, one can see that they eat hawthorn all by themselves when they have health problems or are feeling unwell. In case of laminitis or navicular disease, hawthorn can always be given to supplement other medical procedures. When it's very hot during the summer, old ponies and horses can be given a small daily dose of hawthorn to bolster their circulation. Colic and other illnesses also, can always be treated with hawthorn in addition to other therapies. You will soon find out that the horses are more alert and feel better.

IN USE

If you are a keen herb collector, take a handful of leaves, buds or berries (around 10 g) and prepare as below.

> USED INTERNALLY

Hawthorn can be prepared as an infusion, and then poured over food. My horses love it especially as a solution in alcohol. Hawthorn drops drizzled on bread or sugar can be fed directly, and the active substance is then absorbed quickly via the lining of the mouth. Do not forget: in very old horses especially, hawthorn should always be given over a long period.

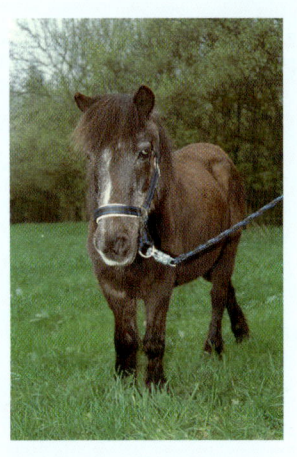

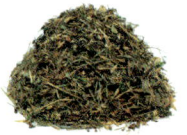

Hay flowers   *Flores graminis*

The origins

> For tense
muscles
> For cramp,
colic and
lumbago
> A good food
supplement

Anyone who wants to see hay flowers in 'the great outdoors' these days, will have to climb very high up. Genuine hay flowers can only be found in the Alps, where nature is still relatively untouched.

The term 'hay flowers' refers to a large number of flowers that make up a meadow. These always include anemones, arnica, hawkweed and milkwort.

Then there are various grasses, sweet vernal grass, brome, quaking grass and meadow grass. Only when the hay flower mixture exhibits the whole force of the aromatic alpine meadow, does it unfold its full effect.

Medicinal properties

**A TIP FROM
THE VET**

Call the vet immediately at the first sign of colic or lumbago. While waiting for the vet to arrive, you can alleviate your horse's condition with a hay flower bag.

Hay flowers are used in human naturopathy mainly by being dried and kept in a linen bag. The bag is warmed up with steam and placed on the body. A hay flower bag is used for digestive disorders, cramps, gastroenteritis, inflammation of the upper respiratory tract, lower abdominal pain, lumbago, muscular rheumatism and many other complaints. The active substances enter the body through the skin and stimulate the nerves and the connective tissue. Hay flower bags are a simple and cost-effective home remedy. If you don't sleep well, make yourself a small linen pillow and fill it with hay flowers.

Hay flowers for horses

Do you want to make your horses happy? Buy hay flowers, mix them into food and let your horses dream about flower meadows. Hay flowers improve every meal and can enrich the horses' menu all year round, especially in winter. They contain many active ingredients in natural form and upgrade every food ration. Warm hay flower bags too, so popular with people, help

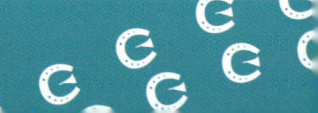

horses with many ailments, for example tense muscles and cramp in the event of colic and lumbago.

IN USE

> USED INTERNALLY

Hay flowers are contained in many food mixtures and herbal supplements. However, you can also buy them in dried form, prepare a tea or mix them into food.

> USED EXTERNALLY

You can make a hay flower bag yourself. Simply sew one out of a piece of linen and fill it with hay flowers. Naturally, for the back of a horse it needs to be sufficiently large. Hay flowers should not be older than one year, after that they lose their effect. Seed mixtures are available commercially, and you can sow your own little herbal meadow in the pasture.

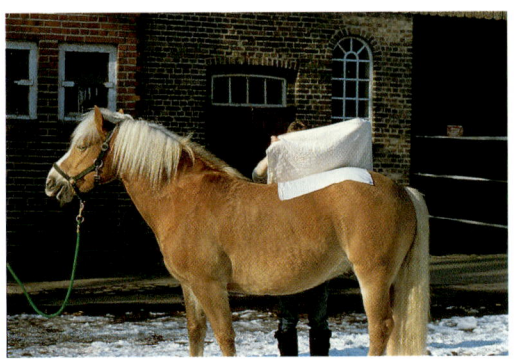
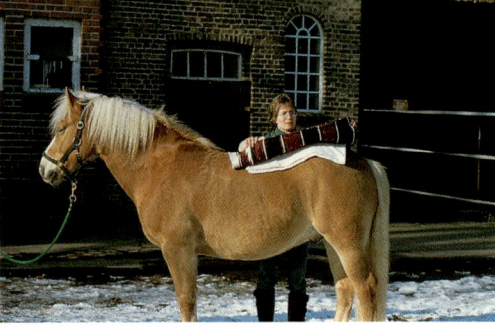

A warm hay flower bag is a boon for tense muscles.

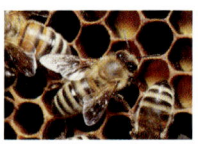

Honey

The origins

Honey means healing power and luxury food in one. The first evidence that humans collected honey goes back to prehistory. The ancient Greeks and the Germanic tribes used honey to make mead, an intoxicating drink. But its healing properties were also discovered early on. Many peoples valued honey as a remedy for wounds and used it for ailments of the respiratory tract and the lungs.

Medicinal properties

Honey has many interesting properties. Anyone who takes it only as a sweetener finds that honey is sweeter than the same amount of sugar, and furthermore contains a whole number of valuable ingredients. Using

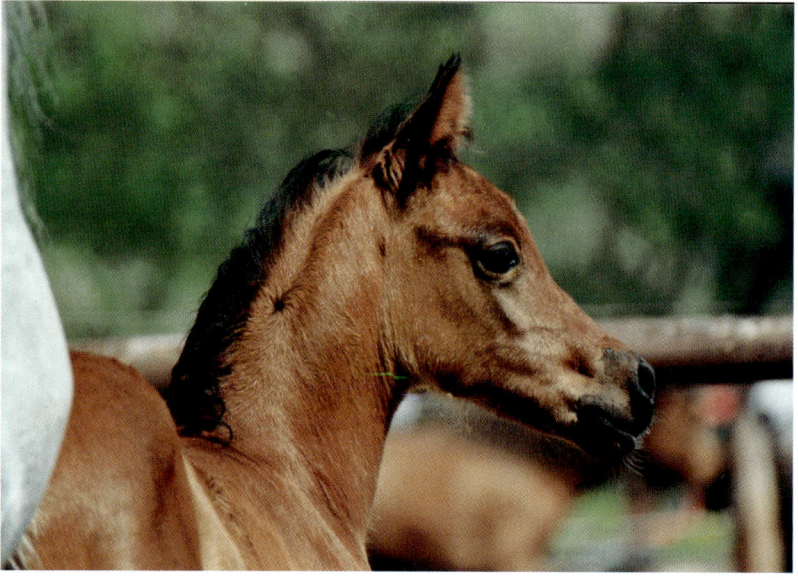

The Arabs gave their foals honey.

honey instead of sugar protects the pancreas and supplies the body with wonderful substances. Honey has an antimicrobial action and is an excellent remedy for wounds, including for inflammations of the oral and gastric mucosa. The most important ingredients in honey are the flavonoids, fructose and glucose, enzymes, B-group vitamins, trace elements, minerals and a hormone-like substance. Since listing all the properties of honey would fill several pages, let's mention only a few. Honey revitalises, strengthens nerves and the immune system, promotes digestion, helps with sleep disorders and restlessness, improves blood circulation in the coronary vessels, and has an antibacterial and anti-inflammatory effect. Honey protects against tumours and can help hold back the years. It can be mixed with many medicinal herbs and improves both their efficacy and taste. You can prepare a universal health elixir from the following ingredients: fruit vinegar/cider vinegar, honey, lemon and garlic. Taken daily, this drink will prevent many ailments.

Honey for horses

All the benefits described in the previous section apply to horses also. They like honey as a treat, and do not refuse even bitter medicine when sweetened with honey. The Arabs used to add honey when feeding foals. Since honey is an excellent remedy for wounds, it is popular for external use also. It can be applied to burns, small grazes and old scars. Honey is also thought to be an antibiotic. If your vet regards it as necessary to give antibiotics, you can invigorate your horse by adding honey. Old and weak animals in particular renew their strength with honey.

IN USE

Try to obtain honey produced locally, and if you know the beekeeper so much the better. Imported honey may be cheap, but may come from contaminated hives. Different kinds of honey should be taken for different ailments. For colds: eucalyptus, fir tree or wildflower honey. As a tonic: lime blossom honey. For horses as for humans, the best preventive against illness is to take cider vinegar with honey every day.

> DOSAGE

Take 2 tablespoons honey with 2 tablespoons cider vinegar and 200 ml water daily.

> USED INTERNALLY

Dilute honey with cider vinegar and water and mix into food, or just add straight honey.

> USED EXTERNALLY

Apply honey to wounds or scars.

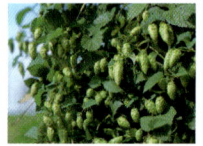

Hops   *Humulus lupulus*

The origins

> Has a calming effect on nervous horses
> Helps with flatulence and digestive disorders

Hops are popular not only with lovers of good beer. Wild hops can be found in shrubs and woods near bodies of water. Hops are cultivated mainly in Europe, but are also planted in northern and central Asia. Their cone-like inflorescence is used both medically and in making beer. Cultivated hops are propagated through rootstock segments. You can try planting them in the garden. Their blossoms and leaves are delightfully decorative.

Medicinal properties

Hops are famous for their calming effect, but they have other benefits also. Their blossoms contain bitter substances, tannins and essential oils, combined in the form of lupulin. This substance is antiseptic, antispasmodic, enhances appetite (as we can see with beer), promotes digestion and relieves pain. Hops can develop their beneficial effects both internally and externally. They go together superbly with other medicinal plants, and often are mixed with balm, valerian, lavender and similar sedatives and analgesics. A herbal pillow filled with hops and lavender ensures restorative sleep.

> ### A TIP FROM THE VET
>
> Scientists have discovered hormonally-active substances in hop blossoms. Therefore the plant is unsuitable for studs and breeding mares.

Hops for horses

In horses, it is primarily the calming and stomach-friendly effects of hops that are helpful. Try to soothe your skittish, tetchy or restless horse with hop tea or tonic. Are you going on a long and unfamiliar journey with your horse? Then treat it for a few days beforehand to hop, valerian and lavender tea. Shortly before going in the box, trickle a few drops of Bach flower rescue remedy into its mouth, and rider and horse will be able to enjoy the trip in peace and quiet.

Hop and chamomile blossoms are a tried and tested remedy for flatulence and digestive disorders. You can add the blossoms to food fresh, dried and powdered or as an infusion.

IN USE

> #### > USED INTERNALLY
>
> Many commercial herbal mixtures for horses contain hops. Their use depends on the specific type. Hop tea is available loose in bulk and in bags, often as a mixture for infusion with valerian and balm.

Single hop blossoms are also available. They are steeped in hot water and after 15 minutes passed through a tea strainer. Then the infusion with the blossoms can be poured over food.

We have a very temperamental warmblood who gets mightily excited over everything new and unfamiliar. He becomes especially difficult when he sees many horses coming towards him. I have now prescribed him a course of infusions. He is given a daily infusion of St John's wort, valerian and hops. Now we just need to wait patiently for the next tournament season.

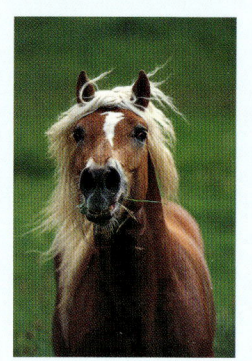

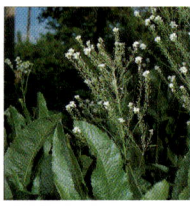

Horseradish   *Armoracia rusticana*

The origins

> Helps to get rid of worms as a supplement to veterinary treatment
> Improves the general condition
> Helps against windgalls

Once again it was St. Hildegard of Bingen who extolled the benefits of the horseradish. It was used even then to alleviate fever and flu, and as a preventive measure against coughs, colds and hoarseness. Horseradish grows in the wild in eastern Europe, Great Britain and the USA, but is now cultivated everywhere. The roots can be collected in the autumn for medicinal purposes. The leaves can be picked at any time.

Medicinal properties

Horseradish is a popular condiment that makes many dishes tastier. Its medicinal benefits should not be underestimated. Horseradish contains a natural antibiotic, allyl isothiocyanate, which attacks fungi and bacteria. Horseradish promotes the secretion of bile, thus making food more digestible and facilitating the digestion of fat. It is mildly laxative, stimulating and anthelmintic. Its stimulating, blood circulation-boosting effect is noticeable even in small quantities. Horseradish poultices alleviate neuralgia and rheumatism.

Horseradish for horses

Horseradish is not a substitute for worming treatment, but should always be given to supplement such treatment or from time to time as an anthelmintic remedy. It improves the appetite of horses too, and stimulates all organ functions. Horses become lively and alert, and it can significantly improve their general condition when suffering from infections. In her book *A Modern Horse Herbal*, Hilary Page Self recommends it for stubborn windgalls.

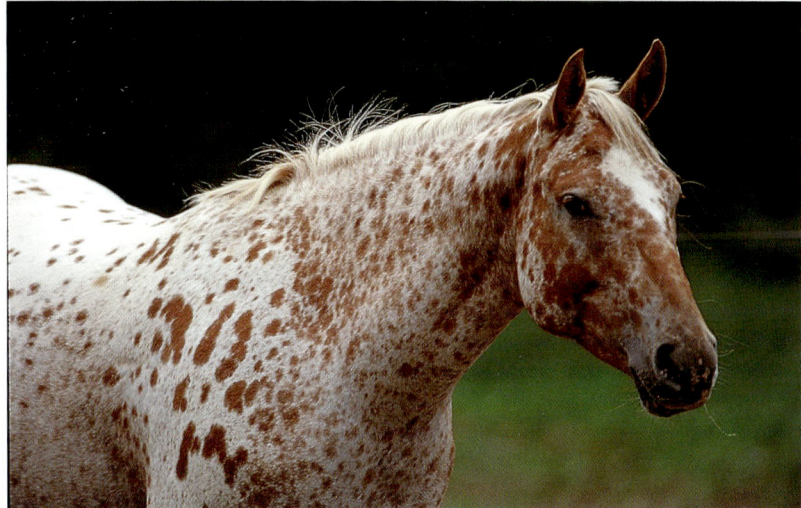

The appetite of horses who are off their food improves with horseradish.

IN USE

Horseradish can be grown in the garden quite easily. Horses like the leaves and also the powdered roots.

> USED INTERNALLY

Like many other herbs, fresh or dried horseradish is added to food. Naturally, you can also buy it everywhere as a condiment.

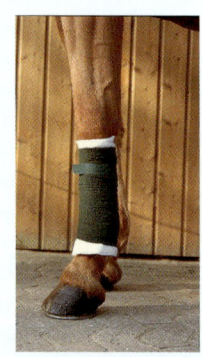

Iceland moss   *Cetrania islandica*

The origins

> Alleviates
irritation in
bronchitis
> Acts as an
antispasmodic
in colic
> Serves
for general
invigoration

The name Iceland moss is incorrect, since this leafless and rootless plant is a lichen, not a moss. It grows on poor, barren soils, in open woods and on moors. It is prevalent mainly at high latitudes in northern Europe, North America, northern Asia and even in the Antarctic. For the animals of the north, Iceland moss is an important food and medicinal plant.

Medicinal properties

Iceland moss is used in various medical conditions. Lichen acids, bitter substances, mucilage and carbohydrates are the most important ingredients. The medicinal properties are antiseptic, appetite-promoting, antispasmodic and emollient. Its anti-emetic benefits are utilised in travel sickness and nausea in general. In weak or sickly people, the digestive glands are stimulated and the appetite boosted. Coughs and lung diseases too, respond positively to Iceland moss.

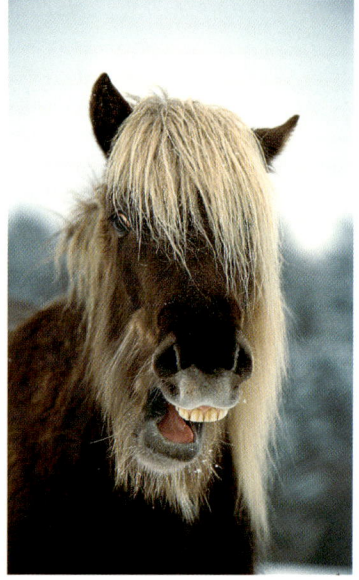

Winter is a time when many horses cough.

Iceland moss for horses

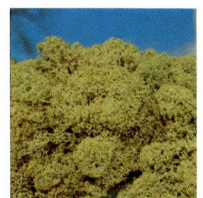

Iceland moss is popular for general invigoration of horses. It is a proven anti-irritant in catarrh of the upper respiratory tract. It has an antispasmodic and balancing effect after colic and in horses that tend to suffer from gastro-intestinal problems. Because of its slightly bitter flavour, it is advisable to sweeten the infusion with a little honey. A popular mixture for coughs or bronchitis consists of Iceland moss, marsh mallow, fennel and thyme.

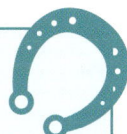

IN USE

Ready-made products and herbal mixtures for horses contain Iceland moss if they are to be effective against coughs and bronchitis. This herbal remedy is also found in restorative tonics. Infusions and dried lichen are available commercially. Because of the flavour, it is advisable to dupe your horse with the aroma of other herbs. All herbal cough remedies and honey, naturally including cider vinegar, are suitable for improving the taste and for reinforcing the positive effect.

> DOSAGE

Feed up to 50 g herbal mixture daily.

> USED INTERNALLY

Add to food a herbal mixture with a tablespoon of honey and a tablespoon of cider vinegar, or make an infusion sweetened with honey and pour it over the food.

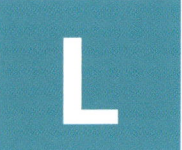

L

Lady's mantle

Alchemilla vulgaris

The origins

> Helps in conjunctivitis
> Alleviates eczema and coat problems
> Effective for mouth inflammation
> Has blood-cleansing properties

In the Middle Ages, lady's mantle was regarded as a miracle remedy. It was supposed to restore virginity, also beauty lost due to age or motherhood. However far-fetched these attributes, lady's mantle really is very useful. It grows all over Europe in grassland, meadows and at the margins of woods. The whole plant with the exception of the root is used for medicinal purposes.

Medicinal properties

Lady's mantle contains organic acids, tannins, resin and saponins, and is an astringent, anti-inflammatory, soothing, antispasmodic and wound-healing remedy. It is beneficial for gastrointestinal disorders, especially diarrhoea and flatulence, for poorly healing wounds and for coughs. In earlier times it was prescribed for gynaecological problems, including in the menopause.

IN USE

> USED INTERNALLY

Lady's mantle can be poured as a tea over food or mixed with other kinds of tea.

> USED EXTERNALLY

Washes and poultices are good for the skin, eyes and poorly healing wounds. For mouth and throat inflammation, mix sage and lady's mantle and rinse the horse's mouth carefully.

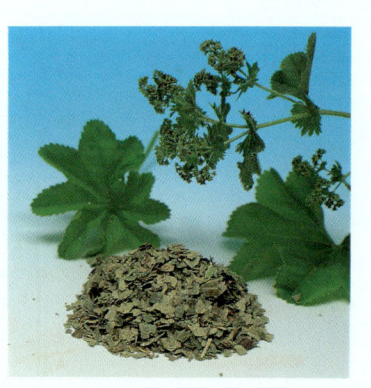

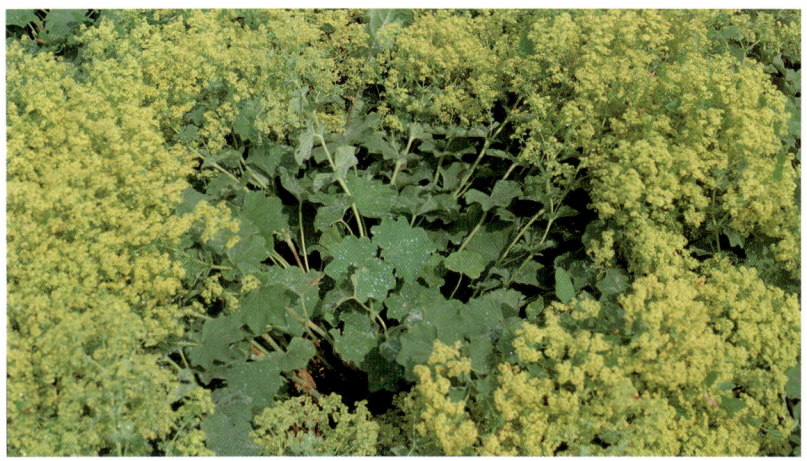

Lady's mantle for horses

For our horses we use lady's mantle internally and externally. In the spring as a blood-cleansing tea, it works well when mixed with nettle. In mild cases of diarrhoea it regulates digestion and soothes the stomach. Externally, lady's mantle is a remedy for conjunctivitis, which especially in the summer occurs often in grazing horses because of the numerous flies. Thanks to its antipruritic properties, it is recommended in combination with fruit vinegar for eczema and other skin and coat problems. It is also beneficial for mouth and throat inflammation.

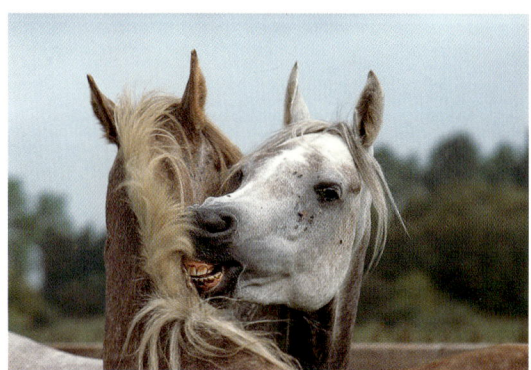

In the summer, grazing horses often have eye and coat problems because of flies.

> Repels flies
> Calms
nervous
horses
> First aid for
insect bites

Lavender

Lavandula officinalis

The origins

Anyone who has ever been on holiday in the south of France can remember the wonderful blue lavender fields, a feast for the eyes and nose. As with so many other plants, the first records can be found in the writings of St. Hildegard of Bingen. Lavender was recommended in the 12th century against cramps, dizziness and mouth ulcers and to fortify the brain. It is at home around the Mediterranean, but has established itself in our gardens, especially in combination with roses (it repels aphids). It is encountered only rarely in the wild as a garden escapee, but in Provence it is planted over large areas for the production of lavender oil.

Medicinal properties

Lavender's essential oils are well-known. It also contains tannins and bitter substances. Its exceptionally calming effect is appreciated in teas and bath salts. It is the most reliable remedy for sleep disorders and restlessness. Lavender promotes the production of bile and is beneficial in case of stomach cramps and other digestive complaints.

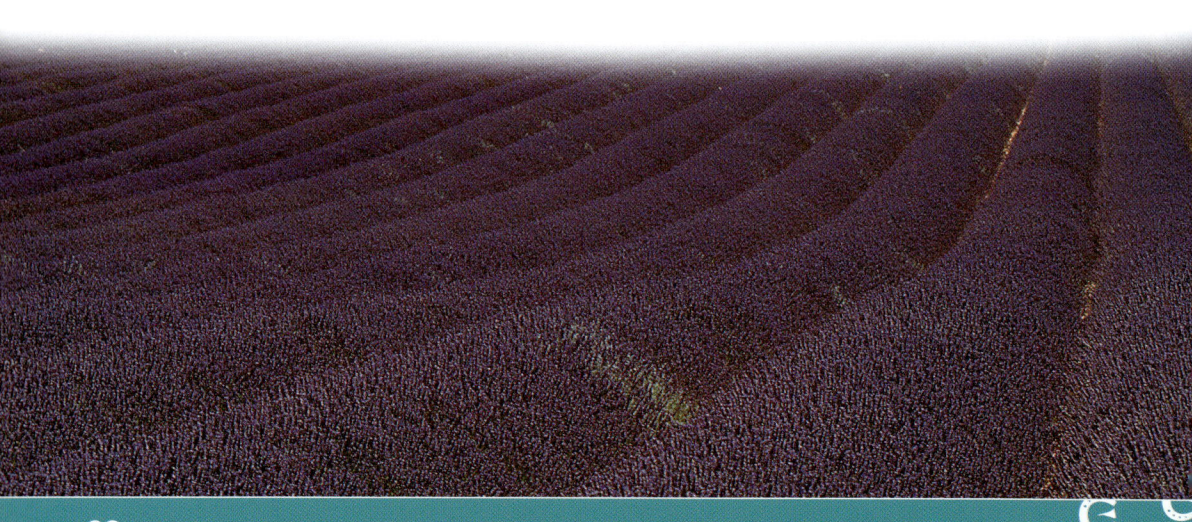

Externally, it helps to treat insect bites, wounds, scalp ringworm, lice infestations and rheumatism.

It is contained in many natural insect repellents.

Lavender for horses

Lavender blossoms can be draped all around the stable in order to keep it free from flies. In combination with garlic its action is even more intensive and it gets rid of the smell of garlic. Lavender keeps moths away from blankets and other horse equipment. Lavender oil is calming to excited, nervous horses just as it is to humans. It is analgesic, antibacterial and promotes the growth of new cells. Since it is very mild, it can even be applied straight to the skin in small quantities. Lavender oil offers quick relief from insect bites.

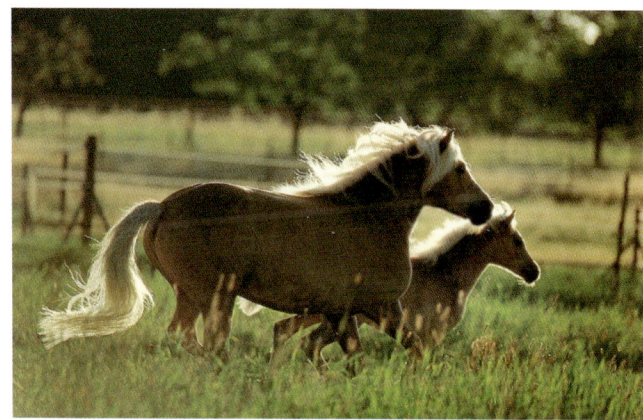

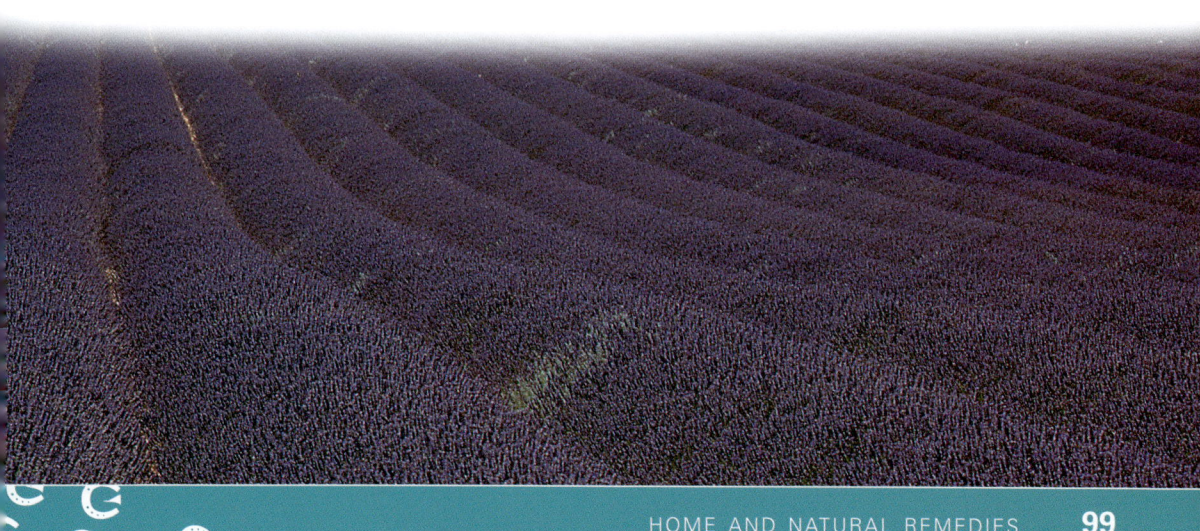

IN USE

Lavender oil is widely available. It mixes well with other oils, for example tea tree oil. Lavender oil makes any combination of oils gentler and milder. Lavender blossoms from the garden are dried and stored carefully.

> USED INTERNALLY

Many food mixtures nowadays contain lavender.

Lavender blossom tea can be combined with many other herbs or tea varieties.

> USED EXTERNALLY

Lavender is contained in many ointments, sprays and lotions. For a calming lavender oil inhalation, it makes sense to prepare a mixture with other oils.

Summer eczema mixtures should contain lavender to repel midges and mosquitoes.

> Calming effect on the respiratory tract and digestive system
> Anti-inflammatory effect benefits the lining of the mouth and throat
> First aid for bronchitis

Lime tree and lime blossom

Tilia cordata –
Tilia platyphyllos

The origins

The stunningly beautiful lime or linden tree can grow up to 30 metres tall. In Germanic mythology it was dedicated to Freya, the goddess of love and marriage. According to legend, it protects against evil spirits and witches. Even today we can sometimes still find, in old unchanged villages, the original linden tree under which people used to meet each other. Many folk songs are dedicated to it, and when it displays its pale green leaves in late spring we know that summer is not far behind.

Medicinal properties

In folk medicine, lime blossom tea is a tried and tested home remedy. Mixed with elderflower, almost everyone has drunk it at one time or another for a cold or a fever. The essential oil, farnesol, is used in natural cosmetics due to its calming effect and unique fragrance. Glycosides, flavonoids and mucilage are other ingredients important in natural medicine. Lime blossom tea has an antispasmodic effect and helps alleviate coughs and bronchitis. Furthermore, these ingredients exert a balancing influence on the digestive system. They have a very powerful calming effect and encourage bile production. Lime blossom tea with honey is a perfect antidote to a hectic day.

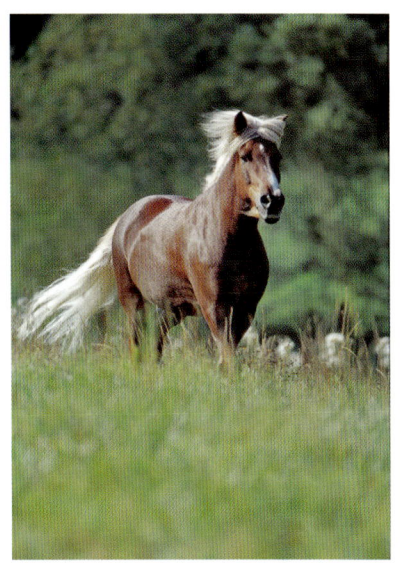

Fresh air and pasture are the best contributors to health.

Lime blossoms for horses

Naturally, we use the anti-irritant, cough-alleviating, calming effect on the respiratory tract and the sensitive digestive system of horses also. In acute or chronic bronchitis, lime blossoms are an especially welcome and valuable supplementary treatment. When you put together a herbal mixture for inhalation, you must not forget lime blossoms. The powerful anti-inflammatory action benefits the mouth's mucous lining and the throat, including in the event of a dry cough caused, for example, by a high level of dust.

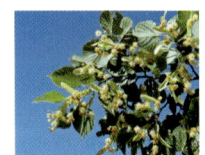

IN USE

> DOSAGE

Once a day 30–50 g blossom infusion as a tea or decoction.

> ## USED INTERNALLY

Regular use fortifies the immune system during the cold season. Most ponies and horses like the flavour, therefore the tea with the blossoms can simply be added to food. Moreover, this binds the dust in food which in turn benefits the mucous linings and respiratory tract.

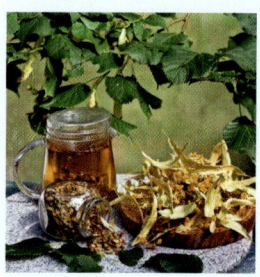

> ## USED EXTERNALLY

For external inflammation you can also try washing with lime blossom tea or decoction.

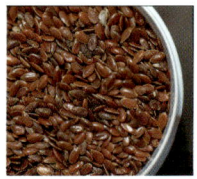

Linseed   *Linum usitatissimum*

The origins

> Strengthens
the digestive
system
> Fortifies
after illness
> Benefits
the change of
coat
> Promotes
a shiny coat
and strong
hooves

Flax is one of the world's oldest cultivated plants, used as far back as approximately 30,000 years ago in the Caucasus as a source of fibres and food and for medicinal purposes. There is documented planting by many ancient peoples around 3,000 BC in China and India.

Flax is described as a remedy in the Ayurveda, the ancient Hindu system of medicine. The Chinese used the plant for intractable constipation and to combat early ageing and grey hair. It also served as a general tonic. Today, flax is cultivated in southern and central Europe.

Medicinal properties

The natural healing powers of flax derive from its seeds. Linseed tastes slimy and oily but has no odour, and it contains a range of different ingredients: mucilage, pectin and up to 40% oil, also proteins, lignans, sugar and sterols.

The seed oil gains its value from the linolenic acid it contains. The clinical efficacy of linseed is manifested in gastritis, indigestion, ulcers and constipation. Its anti-inflammatory properties also help in coughs, hoarseness and urinary tract disorders. Linseed can be relied upon externally also. As a poultice it helps in burns, injuries and abscesses.

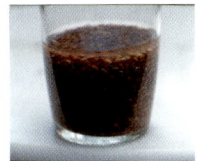

IN USE

Nowadays, of course, you can buy all manner of linseed products ready to use. The mixtures are mostly good and beneficial to horses, but everything comes at a price and those who have the time and want to save money can do the cooking and grinding themselves. The seeds are crushed with an old coffee grinder or nut grinder just before feeding. Before boiling too, they are freshly ground, then afterwards cooled down and mixed with bran, then fed when lukewarm. A treat for your horses after hard work.

> DOSAGE

Once a day mix a handful of freshly ground linseed into concentrated food, or add a handful of cooked linseed to bran and make into mash.

Add a tablespoon of linseed oil to carrots or mix into food.

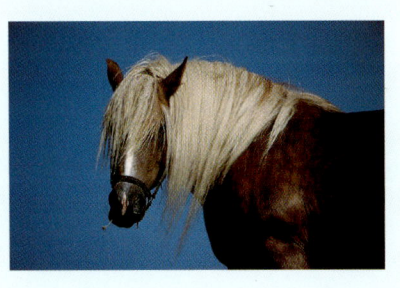

Linseed for horses

No other natural remedy for horses is as well-known as linseed. Even the old stable masters of the past knew countless uses. Every horse owner and stable hand has given his horse linseed in one form or another. Supplementing food with linseed or linseed oil should be a matter of course these days. The horse's digestive system is fortified and stabilised, and it regains its strength more rapidly after colic and other ailments. Following severe colic and a very stressed gastrointestinal tract, give only linseed gruel.

CAUTION
Linseed contains prussic acid and should not be fed in large quantities.

There is a positive effect on the muscles. The change of coat proceeds faster and with fewer problems if linseed is given regularly. Mares after foaling have earned a good mash. Linseed oil may well be the most suitable oil for horses: ordinary cooking oils are difficult for horses to digest, since horses have no gall bladder. For skin and coat problems you can try a course of linseed oil: the skin will become more elastic and the itching may be relieved. Linseed poultices are a proven remedy for lumbago, colic and hoof ulcers.

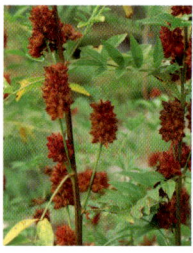

Liquorice   *Glycyrrhiza glabra*

The origins

> Beneficial for respiratory disorders
> Antispasmodic action
> Boosts hormone production

Liquorice is a plant of Mediterranean regions, but its subspecies occur worldwide. The ancient Egyptians were once again the first who were familiar with its medicinal use. But in Greece too, it was known for its sweet flavour and its soothing properties. Today, liquorice is added to medications and cough remedies to improve the taste. The root is the part most utilised, sometimes the leaves also.

Medicinal properties

Liquorice is not only a coveted sweet for children and adults. It consists primarily of the thickened sap of the plant, which contains sugar, tannin, flavonoids and glycyrrhetic acid. It promotes expectoration in coughs and bronchitis, alleviates coughs and is an antispasmodic. The blood-cleansing and digestion-promoting properties of liquorice are valued also. Even the cosmetics industry makes good use of its refreshing and softening effect.

Liquorice for horses

Let us practise what the North American natives used to do. They rubbed their horses' chafed areas of skin with liquorice leaves, which may be an option for dealing with summer eczema.

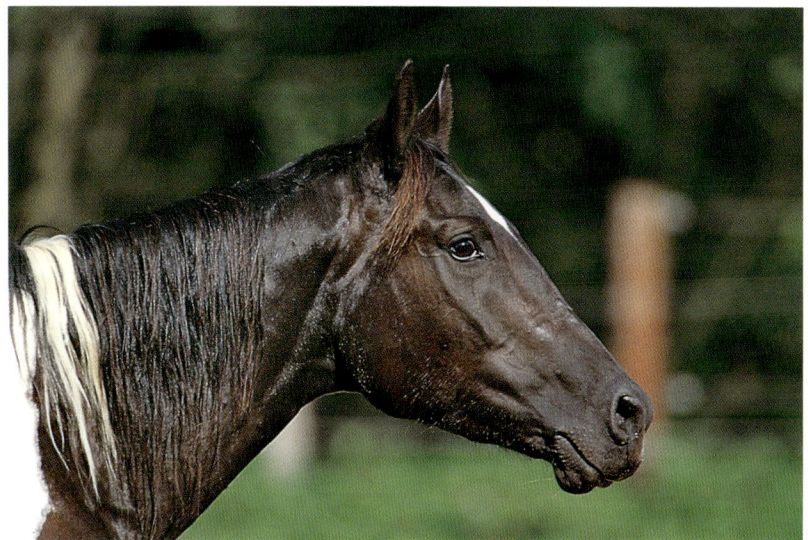

Horses like eating liquorice – and it helps alleviate respiratory disorders.

Unfortunately, horses often suffer from respiratory disorders. Liquorice root acts as an expectorant, alleviates irritation and fights inflammation.

Gastritis and liver damage can also benefit from treatment with small doses of liquorice. It has been demonstrated that liquorice boosts hormone production and increases the fertility of mares. Pregnant mares should not be given liquorice.

IN USE

You will not need to coax your horses to take liquorice, since they love the flavour. These days, it is often added to herbal mixtures, natural cough remedies and mixed feed. Liquorice is available as an infusion, thickened juice and ready-made cough syrup. All these can be given to horses.

> DOSAGE

Give 20 g dried roots daily. Cough syrup should be given according to the dosage instructions.

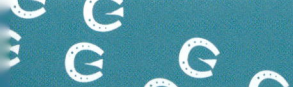

M

Marigold

Calendula officinalis

The origins

Once again it was St. Hildegard of Bingen who in the 12th century first described the marigold. It was known in the Middle Ages as a remedy for digestion complaints, wild animal bites and eczema. Marigold blooms worldwide, but comes originally from the Mediterranean region. Here it is a popular, beautiful garden plant. We use the healing properties of the petals or of the whole flower.

Medicinal properties

> Belongs in every stable
> For small wounds
> For mouth and eye inflammation

Almost everyone is familiar with marigold in the form of ointment, and it has become a popular folk remedy. The substances it contains, including essential oils, flavonoids, carotenoids and saponins, make it especially useful for healing wounds and for treating many skin problems. It is an antibacterial, antifungal and strong anti-inflammatory remedy. Its ointments, tinctures

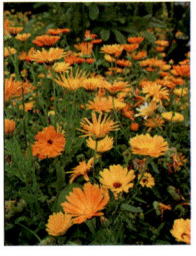

Small wounds are treated quickly with marigold ointment.

and extracts are suitable for treating all kinds of injuries and inflammations, including in the mouth and the eyes. Internally, marigold is beneficial in digestive complaints, stomach ulcers, irritable states and restlessness.

Marigold for horses

Marigold ointment or tincture belongs in every stable's medicine cabinet. Minor wounds that our horses may suffer in the stable and pasture can be treated with marigold. In case of more serious injuries, for example heavy bruising, you should of course always call a vet or natural health professional. Small burns and ulcers respond well to marigold. In particular, mouth and eye inflammation can be flushed with the tincture or a compress applied.

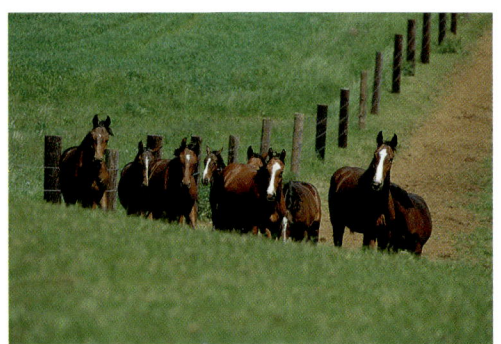

Marigold is beneficial for stomach complaints and urinary tract infections, and also helps in liver disorders. If your horse suffers from fungal infections, malanders or thrush, make an infusion or decoction for rinsing. Marigold can be mixed with other medicinal herbs to treat summer eczema.

IN USE

> USED INTERNALLY

Collect the yellow blossoms of marigold carefully in your garden. They can be fed to horses in the usual dosage, fresh or dried. If you have marigold in the meadow, your animals will eat it very quickly. From experience I know that ponies and goats leave nothing standing. Marigold blossoms have to be dried very carefully, preserving the yellow colour as far as possible.

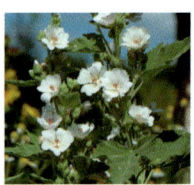

Marsh mallow   *Althaea officinalis*

The origins

> To prevent
cramp colic
> For coughs,
bronchitis and
an irritated
respiratory
tract
> For skin
problems and
inflammation

Charlemagne issued an ordinance as far back as the 8th century that the
marsh mallow should be grown as a medicinal plant. Originally, the marsh
mallow was at home in southern Europe and Asia, but it has long since
spread across Europe, Asia and Australia. Its roots and leaves are used internally and externally to treat many ailments.

Medicinal properties

It is especially the mucilage contained within it which makes the marsh
mallow an anti-inflammatory medicinal plant. But it has even more to offer:
vitamin C, carbohydrates, minerals, starch and pectin are responsible for its
cough-alleviating and stomach-friendly effects. Marsh mallow helps with
abscesses, eye inflammations, bladder inflammation, diarrhoea and gum
problems. Its pleasantly-tasting ingredients are frequently contained in
medicines for children. There are no known side-effects.

Marsh mallow for horses

Marsh mallow finds many applications in natural medicine for horses, too. Ground marsh mallow root is a preventive in horses that tend to suffer from cramp colic. Stomach ulcers and gastrointestinal inflammation are affected positively. Marsh mallow leaves and roots are given for coughs, bronchitis and an irritated respiratory tract. They facilitate expectoration and soothe the airways. Externally, marsh mallow is beneficial for skin problems and inflammation.

IN USE

Because of its cough-alleviating and digestion-promoting effects, marsh mallow is added to many food and herbal mixtures and other ready-to-use products. It can also be planted in the garden. However, don't collect it where it grows naturally, since it is a protected plant. It is tasty, and horses eat it readily. To help with a cough, you can add honey.

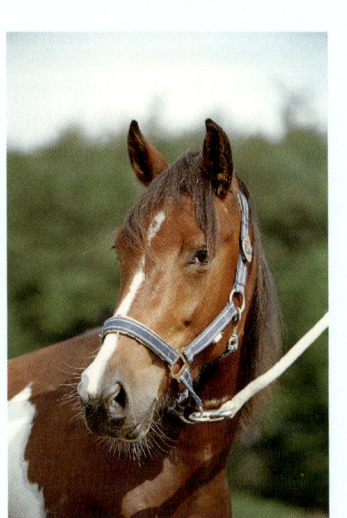

> USED INTERNALLY

Marsh mallow (50 g daily) can be prepared as a tea by adding either hot water (allow to brew for 10 minutes) or cold water (let stand for 1 hour); then pour it over food.

The plant (50 g) or its roots (around 20 g) can also be sprinkled loosely over food.

You can also buy marsh mallow powder and give it once a day as directed (around 15 g).

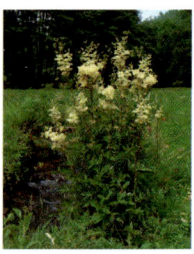

Meadowsweet   *Filipendula ulmaria*

Mead wort

The origins

The medieval botanists were familiar with meadowsweet, but its medical properties were first described in later herbals. It was valued for its gall bladder-cleansing and vesicant effect.

Today it is known mainly for its salicylic acid compounds, the modern painkillers.

Meadowsweet can be found all over Europe and Asia along damp ditches and embankments and in meadows.

Aspirin, which is a salicylic acid compound, derives its name from meadowsweet's Greek name, spinia.

> Helps in
> rheumatism
> Alleviates
> lameness
> Good for
> muscle and
> joint pain
> Good for
> elderly horses

Medicinal properties

In addition to its main active substance, salicylic acid, meadowsweet contains flavonoid compounds, tannins and mineral salts. Its tea extracts are astringent, diuretic, antispasmodic and strongly analgesic.

Meadowsweet is an excellent remedy for gastric and intestinal disorders and helpful in diarrhoea and cramps. Fever and rheumatic pain are alleviated, and its anti-inflammatory effect is manifested to the full in flu, painful limbs and muscles and sciatica. Meadowsweet dilates the blood vessels and fortifies cardiac function.

A TIP FROM THE VET

Never boil up: only pour boiling water on the blossoms. Caution in case of hypersensitivity to salicylic compounds!

Meadowsweet for horses

Meadowsweet has long had an established place in equine naturopathy.

It is especially the effect on the sensitive digestive organs of horses that is emphasised time and again. Old horses in particular often suffer from rheumatism, their cardiac function may need to be assisted and their gastrointestinal tract has become more sensitive. This is where meadowsweet displays its wide-ranging effect on all these ailments.

Externally, meadowsweet can be used for wound healing and pain relief.

The active substances in meadowsweet are recommended in particular for colds and in blood-cleansing teas. They are regarded as diuretic, and can be given as an infusion without concern about side-effects.

IN USE

> USED INTERNALLY

The blossoms are utilised medicinally, less often the roots. The usual form of administration is as an infusion. Horses suffering from the relevant complaints should have the infusion poured over their food several times a day, but you can also mix dried blossoms into the oats. Meadowsweet is excellent for mixing with other herbal teas, since it enhances the effect of other remedies. It is offered as part of many ready-made herbal mixtures.

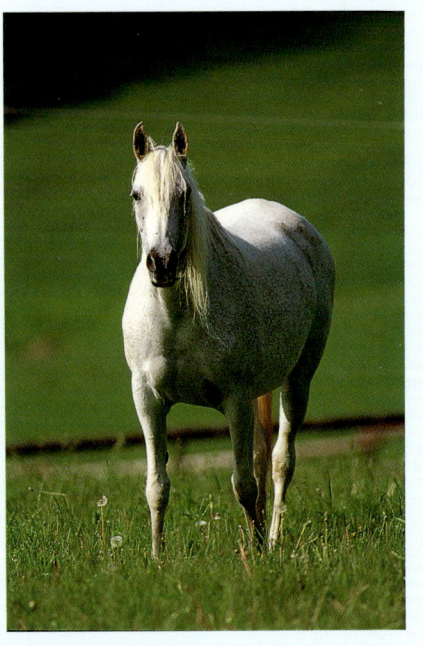

> USED EXTERNALLY

Use a strong infusion externally for wound healing or rheumatism.

When using a decoction or infusion to treat wounds, strain out the blossoms and dab the wound carefully with the liquid only.

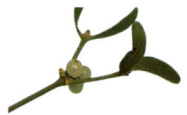

Mistletoe

Viscum album

The origins

The approximately 1,400 species of mistletoe grow on trees and are mainly prevalent in tropical regions. Their medicinal use can be traced back to the fifth century BC. Hildegard of Bingen too, recommended mistletoe against asthma and epilepsy. Rudolf Steiner, the founder of anthroposophy, developed an anti-cancer treatment method using mistletoe. Nowadays, mistletoe still plays a part in naturopathy in the treatment of tumours.

Medicinal properties

The medicinally efficacious parts of mistletoe are the young leaves, fresh or dried. Mistletoe is supposed to inhibit tumour growth and stimulate the immune system due to the flavonoids, resins, alkaloids and mucilage contained within it. The heart's performance is boosted, blood pressure is decreased and the balance of the nervous system improved. In the treatment of the ageing heart, mistletoe has gained a reputation in many combined preparations. Rheumatic disorders also respond positively to mistletoe.

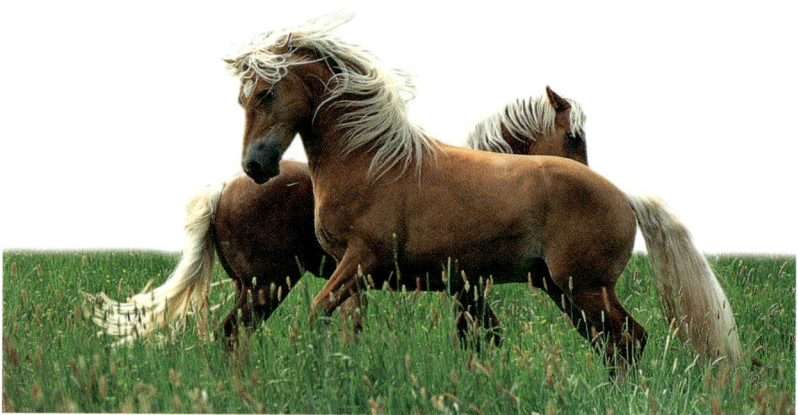

Mistletoe is a fortifying tonic and strengthens the cardiovascular system.

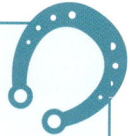

IN USE

> USED INTERNALLY

Injections must only be given by an experienced therapist, vet or natural health practitioner. In homeopathy, Viscum album may be given in the form of drops. Mistletoe tea is widely available and can be given to horses with their food. However, you can also collect mistletoe yourself, dry it and prepare an infusion from it. Mistletoe tea can be given over a prolonged period, and it mixes well with other types of tea. Ready-made preparations are available from suppliers of equine products.

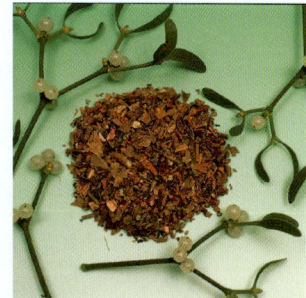

> DOSAGE

Give around 50 g daily as an infusion over food. Homeopathic dosage is according to the vet's directions.

Mistletoe for horses

For older horses in particular, mistletoe is regarded as a tonic for the cardio-vascular system. Horses exhausted after a long illness or excessive training can be fortified with mistletoe extract. A four-week course of treatment against osteoarthritis can benefit any elderly horse. For tumour and cancer therapy, mistletoe must be injected by an experienced vet. But supplementing this with the tea will not do any harm and can have a supportive effect. In homeopathy, mistletoe under its name Viscum album can be of great benefit in bronchitis, broken wind, tumours, osteoarthritis and in treating the ageing heart.

> Helps in
hormonal
disorders
> Promotes
oestrus

Monk's pepper

Chaste tree

Vitex agnus castus

The origins

Monk's pepper has been known as a medicinal plant since the 4th century. It is found mainly in the northern Mediterranean region and in central Asia. Monk's pepper really does derive its name from monks: the plant is supposed to suppress the sex drive, therefore in earlier times nuns and monks had it placed in front of the door when they entered the convent or monastery.

Medicinal properties

Monk's pepper has been tested thoroughly in recent years. It exercises a significant regulating effect on hormone production. Its active substances – iridoids and flavonoids – have a positive influence on menstruation disorders and swollen breasts associated with the cycle. Use is made of its seeds and fruit, available commercially in the form of drops.

IN USE

> DOSAGE

Add 15 g monk's pepper over food for four to eight weeks. Do not feed monk's pepper during gestation.

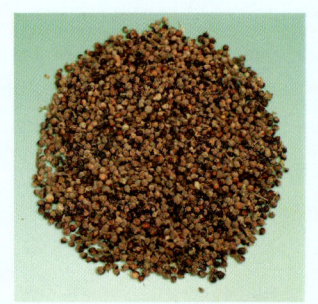

> USED INTERNALLY

If the mare does not come on heat, the plant can regulate and stabilise the cycle.

Monk's pepper for horses

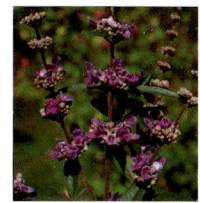

Stallions, mares and also late geldings can become unpredictable and dangerous due to hormonal fluctuations. I experienced this once in a mare with an excellent disposition. She was lunged carefully and gently, and was attentive and very sweet-natured. During her first oestrus after starting under saddle she turned out to be dangerous and impossible to ride. Hormone treatments brought no change. Unfortunately, at the time I had not yet heard about monk's pepper, which perhaps might have been the solution. The mare was sold for breeding as she was unfit for riding.

If you have problems with your horses that are attributable to hormone balance disorders, talk to your vet and try monk's pepper. In cases involving behavioural problems due to hormonal causes in mares, stallions and geldings, it is always worthwhile to give monk's pepper for four to eight weeks and have a little patience.

Mussel extract   *Glycosaminoglycans*

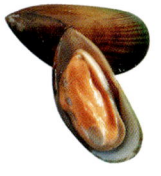

The origins

For generations mussels have been one of the principal food sources of the Maoris, the native inhabitants of New Zealand. Scientists have found that Maoris virtually never suffer from rheumatism, and have traced this phenomenon back to the positive effect of mussel extracts.

Glycosaminoglycans are natural components of the connective tissue, and since 1974 have been used successfully in the treatment of arthritis and osteoarthritis.

> Alleviates painful joints
> Acts preventively in situations of extreme stress
> Helps in tendon injuries

Medicinal properties

Mussel extracts act in particular on the bones, tendons and ligaments. The connective tissue is stabilised and wear is prevented. Rheumatic complaints can be influenced positively, and mobility remains conserved. Faster regeneration is

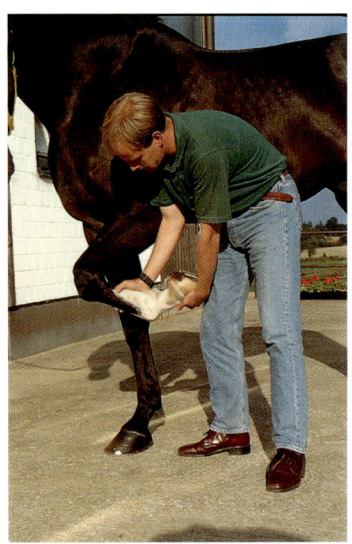

Mussel extract is the right remedy in tendon injuries.

achieved after sports injuries. Metabolic functions can be stimulated and boosted.

Mussel extract for horses

Bones, tendons, ligaments and the connective tissue as a whole are under special stress in horses. Lameness, injured tendons, painful joints and podotrochlear inflammation often follow. Moreover, poor metabolism can lead to rheumatism or excessive wear in the joints.

Mussel extracts stabilise the musculoskeletal apparatus, help to prevent lameness and enhance performance. Trials have shown that mussel extract can not only alleviate joint pain, but also significantly shorten healing times after tendon and joint injuries. It appears to inhibit the formation and release of prostaglandins, acting in this way as an analgesic and anti-inflammatory agent.

Highly physically stressed sport horses should be given mussel extracts regularly. This ensures that they receive an optimal supply of glycosaminoglycans, which are necessary for the metabolism of joints and tendons during intensive work.

Trivial injuries too, which a horse can easily incur during training, heal up quickly and without problems with mussel extracts. In this way more serious tendon damage can be prevented.

A TIP FROM THE VET

In the event of lameness or major medical problems you should of course consult your vet in order to diagnose the extent of the injury. Along with the veterinary procedures you can always give mussel extract.

IN USE

> USED INTERNALLY

Mussel extracts are available from specialist suppliers in many forms. Mostly they are offered as a powder or pellets. Very often they are also combined with other active ingredients. Herbs, algae, vitamins and minerals are ideal for complementing mussel extract.

Prolonged use is important in order to achieve an optimal effect. For problem horses, ongoing feeding is also possible.

Mussel extracts are given with concentrated food according to the appropriate dosage instructions.

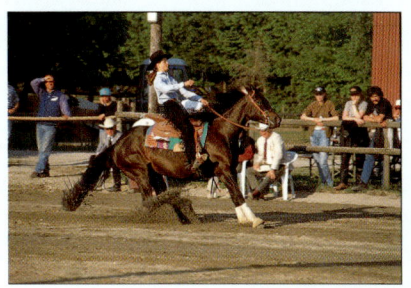

Nettle   *Urtica dioica*

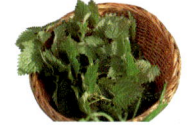

The origins

The nettle may be unloved as a weed, but it is loved as a medicinal plant. As far back as the Middle Ages, people utilised its many benefits. Its fibres were harvested for nettle cloth. Used both internally and externally, its useful properties were greatly valued.

Not only a food plant for butterflies but also a genuine folk medicine, the nettle has now regained its honour. Whipping with a nettle shoot is still practised for sciatica and lumbago. According to the old popular belief, nettle protects against lightning, witches and vermin, and prevents milk and beer turning sour. Because of their particularly high content of leaf pigments, nettles are used for chlorophyll extraction and as a versatile source of a natural green dye.

> Cleanses the blood
> Strengthens the liver
> Invigorates older horses
> Helps in laminitis, rheumatism and summer eczema

Medicinal properties

Naturally, even the nettle is not a wonder drug, but its medicinal effect on many maladies is undisputed. It contains tannins, minerals, vitamins A and C, flavonoids, protein and unsaturated fatty acids. It has an astringent, blood-forming and blood-cleansing effect, and promotes urine and milk production.

Its use, both internally and externally, is tried and tested in anaemia, haemorrhage, diabetes, nosebleeds, hives, oedema, psoriasis and rheumatism.

Because of its tannin content, nettle is also used to combat stomach complaints and diarrhoea. Nettle fruit contains protein, mucilage and lots of unsaturated fatty acids.

Nettle for horses

You can enrich any horse pasture with nettles. Leave them a little room along hedges and fences or under fruit trees. Not only do our horses need them, but so also do numerous butterflies. A course of treatment with nettles is especially beneficial to horses and their riders in the spring. It cleanses the blood and strengthens the liver.

This is particularly important for horses who tend to suffer from laminitis, rheumatism or summer eczema.

When a horse with laminitis is about to go out grazing in the spring, stimulate its blood circulation with nettle tea. Externally, you can rinse the mane and tail with the decoction or tea. Giving nettles regularly to older horses in particular is a wonderful restorative. Furthermore, it helps to ensure a beautiful, silky coat.

IN USE

> USED INTERNALLY

Since horses rarely eat the nettles where they grow, they can simply be mown and dried. Then they no longer sting and are happily eaten by horses. However, once dried you can also chop them into small pieces and mix them into food. Nettle tea is available commercially in many forms. Nettles are also added these days to many kinds of food supplements.

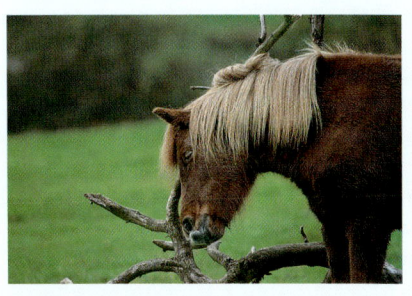

Onion

Allium cepa

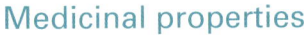

O

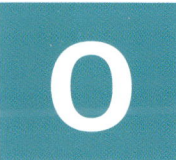

The origins

Onions were popular as much as 5,000 years ago. As today, they were used
as food, condiments and medicinal plants. Onions were grown in medieval
monastery gardens, and their healing properties utilised to treat coughs,
rheumatism and heart disease. Onions come in the widest range of shapes
and colours, but they differ from each other mainly by their odour and flavour. In recent times, science too has become interested in the onion and
has confirmed its health-boosting properties.

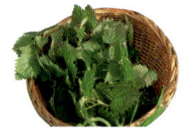

> *Good against
insect bites*
> *Beneficial for
coughs and
bronchitis*
> *In homeopathic
form, helpful in
allergies*

Medicinal properties

The onion is quite similar to garlic, but its odour is a little milder and does
not persist for as long. Onions contain many minerals and trace elements,
a great deal of vitamin C and B-group vitamins, and also flavonoids. Onions
stimulate the appetite and boost the digestion. Their expectorant and anti-
inflammatory properties are beneficial when suffering from coughs and
bronchitis. Regular consumption improves blood fat levels and lowers blood
pressure. Onions are also mildly dehydrating, and lower blood sugar levels

slightly. Raw onions should be eaten to protect against cardiac infarcts and other vascular diseases.

Onion for horses

An onion in the stable is always useful. When sliced, it emits an odour that flies and midges dislike. If nevertheless a horse is bitten, immediately drizzle some onion juice on the affected area: this prevents swelling and itching (also recommended for the rider). A home-made onion syrup benefits sufferers of coughs and bronchitis. A small daily dose of onions wards off the signs of old age and improves the intestinal flora.

Onion poultices are good for pain and inflammations. In homeopathy, Allium cepa is recommended for a running nose and watery eyes, and also for allergies.

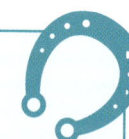

IN USE

Fresh onions are valuable because they contain a plethora of vitamins, but they are still beneficial when dried.

> USED EXTERNALLY

For stings and to repel insects, slice a fresh onion and use the juice, or press the cut side directly against the stung spot.

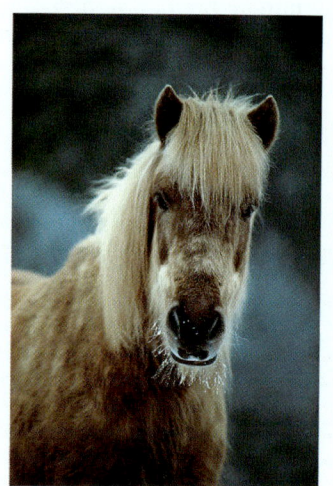

> USED INTERNALLY

You can easily make onion cough syrup yourself. Cut an onion into small pieces (preferably slices) and steep in honey for 24 hours, stirring occasionally. Give a spoonful of this mixture at regular intervals during the day. You can give an onion to eat at the same time. If the horse really dislikes onions, you can strain the broth through a sieve, or mix with fruit vinegar.

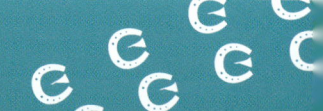

Oregano

Wild marjoram

Origanum vulgare

> Poultices for rheumatic complaints
> Good after long rides
> Good for the digestion

The origins

Oregano is another herb that protects against witches and devils. At least, that is what people believed in the Middle Ages. But even without these magical powers, oregano has many healing properties.

Oregano occurs throughout Europe and is not very choosy about where it grows, but avoids all manured, mown and grazed locations. Unfortunately, therefore, it will not take up residence on a horse pasture. You can, nonetheless, sow it in your organic garden without much difficulty.

Medicinal properties

Oregano is easy to dry, and produces the well-known condiment without which Italian cuisine would be inconceivable.

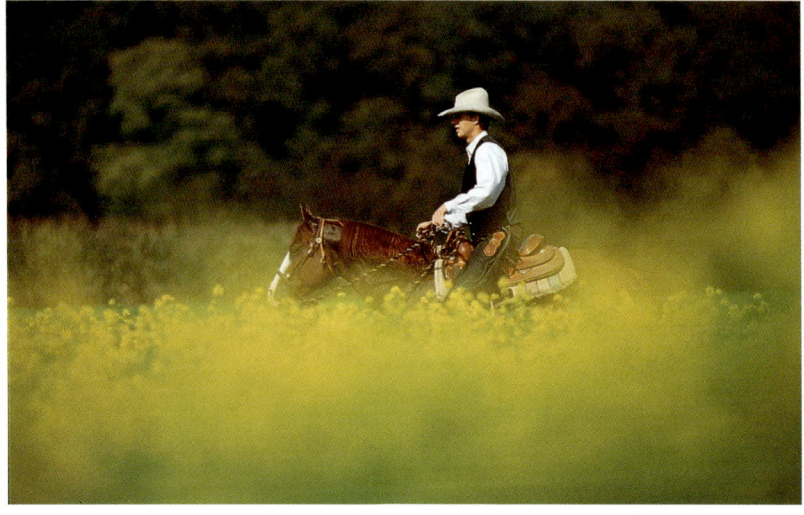

An oregano poultice is soothing and relaxing after a long, strenuous ride.

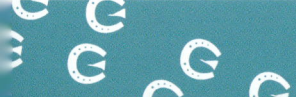

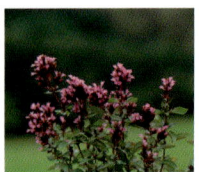

It has a stimulating effect on the nervous system and analgesic properties. Oregano is an antiparasitic, antiseptic, antispasmodic and analgesic remedy and is used to treat asthma. It is beneficial for muscle and rheumatic pain and for tiredness and exhaustion.

Oregano for horses

Oregano can be used in horses both internally and externally. Internally, it has a good effect in particular on the bronchi and on the gastrointestinal system. Externally, a poultice or wash helps with rheumatic complaints and muscle pain.

After over-exertion or excessively long rides, and in cold and wet weather, a warm oregano poultice soothes and relaxes.

IN USE

> USED INTERNALLY

The shoots can be used to make a tasty drink that stimulates the appetite, helps with digestion and alleviates coughs.

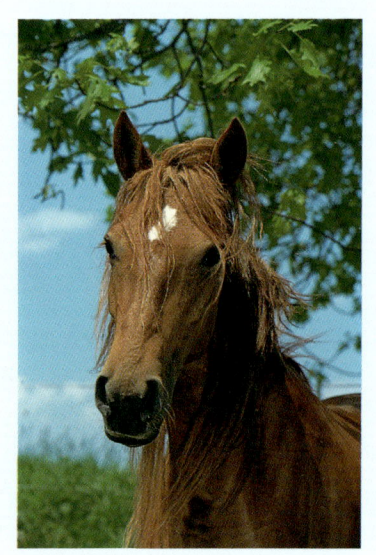

> USED EXTERNALLY

For external use, dry oregano twigs are boiled in water for a few minutes and allowed to infuse for half an hour.

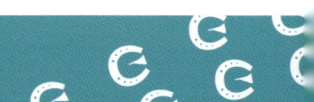

Parsley

Petroselinum crispum

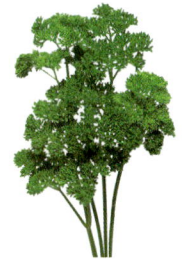

The origins

Parsley is likely to have originated in the Orient. It has been present in herbal gardens since antiquity. The ancient Romans and Greeks loved parsley as a medicinal plant and used it to flavour their dishes. Even today its valuable ingredients, for example its high iron content, mean that parsley is more than just a seasoning herb.

It is important to enjoy parsley while it is as fresh as possible.

During long storage and under the heat of cooking, some of its outstanding substances are lost. Parsley should not be used merely as decoration when serving food: utilise this healthy herb as seasoning for your dishes. If you do not grow parsley yourself, you can buy it fresh, dried or deep-frozen.

> *> Boosts the immune system*
> *> Has a diuretic effect*
> *> Helps to combat anaemia*

Medicinal properties

Parsley is a real powerhouse if we think about the many valuable substances it contains. In addition to essential oils it contains alkaloids, iron, calcium, phosphorus and a lot of vitamins A and C. Five grams of fresh parsley meet the daily requirement of vitamin A, and 30 g that of vitamin C. Parsley detoxifies the body and stimulates many organs. It has an appetite-boosting and blood-cleansing effect. Since parsley contains a great deal of iron and therefore promotes blood production, it is an excellent remedy for those suffering from anaemia. This little herb aids the digestion process, helps

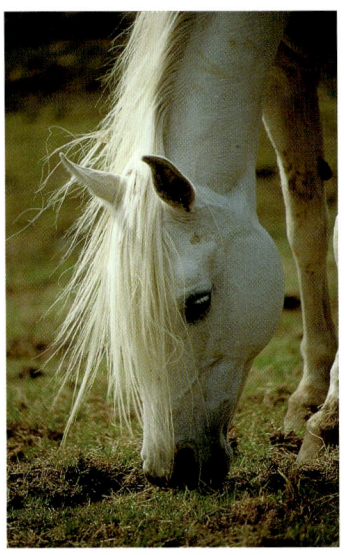

Parsley boosts the appetite.

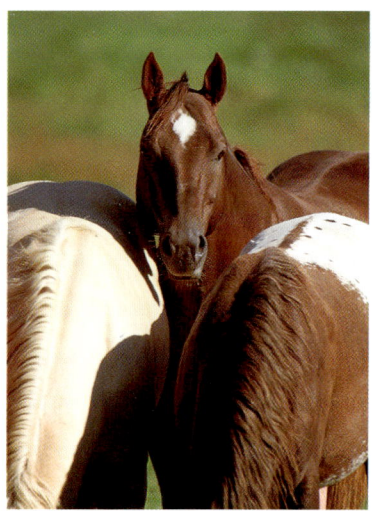

Horses too can sometimes be listless and tired.

the body to break down more rapidly the toxic substances formed as a result of alcohol abuse, and is even supposed to enhance virility. In breastfeeding mothers it stimulates the flow of milk. Externally, parsley has a positive effect on all skin functions and helps in cases of skin blemishes and acne.

Parsley for horses

The high vitamin content of parsley boosts the body's defences. Parsley is also a strong diuretic and can help combat urinary tract infections. It is beneficial in anaemia, rheumatism and digestion problems. Thanks to its many vitamins, parsley makes horses fit and lively. However, it must not be given to pregnant mares because it induces labour.

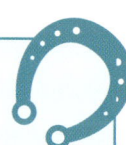

IN USE

Parsley is really easy to grow. If you don't have a garden, use pots on the windowsill. You can buy this popular herb fresh and dried everywhere, even at the supermarket.

> DOSAGE

Fresh parsley has the most intense effect. Your horse may eat three handfuls of parsley per day. If occasionally it grabs a little more in the garden, that too is not a disaster.

The right amount of dried parsley, as with all dried herbs, is about 30 g. Parsley roots can also be fed to horses (two roots per day).

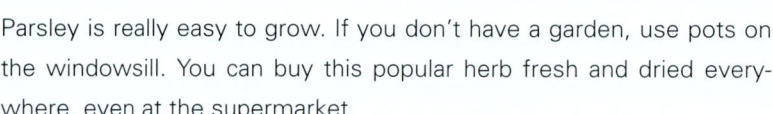

Peppermint

Mentha x piperita

> Preventive effect against colic
> Has an expectorant effect in coughs and bronchitis
> Helps to alleviate insect bites and fungal infections

The origins

Even in antiquity, peppermint was valued as a medicinal plant and for flavouring. Mint plants exist in a wide variety of forms and species, but they are very much alike in their properties. Peppermint grows in nearly all temperate zones around the globe, on humid, humus-rich soils.

IN USE

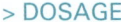

If you want to do something nice for your horses, plant peppermint on the pasture. Horses like eating it and will help themselves. Peppermint can be grown in the garden and even in a flowerpot. Due to the essential oils, fresh peppermint is the most effective compared with dried. Even so, you should dry your peppermint for the winter in bundles and then feed it to the horses regularly. Do you keep a goat in the stable? Treat it to some peppermint, since goats love this herb. If you are unable to grow fresh peppermint, you can buy peppermint tea everywhere. Almost all herbal mixtures and many ready-made food products for horses contain peppermint.

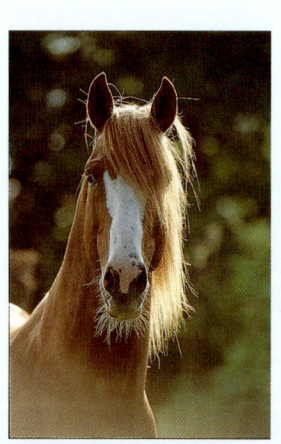

> DOSAGE

Add up to 50 g dried peppermint to food daily or brew a tea.

> USED INTERNALLY

Add fresh or dried peppermint or tea to food.

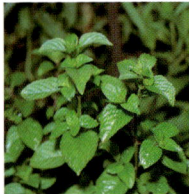

Medicinal properties

The main properties of peppermint derive from its essential oils with menthol compounds and tannins. Peppermint is used internally for colic, gastritis, flatulence and abdominal cramp. In addition, it is an expectorant in coughs and bronchitis. When used for inhalation, it improves nasal breathing and clears the head, for example in migraine. Peppermint is available in many forms: as infusions, inhalations, bath salts, ointments and lozenges. Peppermint tea has no adverse side-effects. Peppermint oil and menthol must never be used in the case of babies and small children.

Peppermint for horses

Horses love the taste of peppermint and do not need a lot of persuasion to accept it. Peppermint makes food more digestible, and calms and relaxes the stomach and intestines. Menthol acts against bacteria and parasites, and the essential oils help to prevent flatulence, colic and even stomach ulcers. Horses that tend to suffer from colic should be given a small daily dose of peppermint or peppermint tea in their food.

You should always think about peppermint when changing the diet, in the spring, the autumn, hay to silage and vice versa. Peppermint inhalations greatly alleviate coughs in horses. Externally, peppermint helps to alleviate insect bites, fungal eczema and the itching of summer eczema. In suckling mares, peppermint helps the udder to return to its normal size once the foal has been weaned.

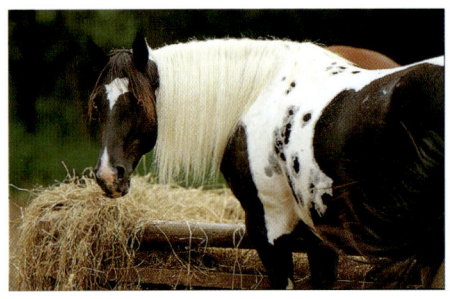

Peppermint helps when changing the diet.

Potatoes   *Solanum tuberosum*

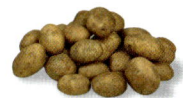

The origins

During the conquest of Peru and Chile, the Spanish came to know the potato as a crop grown by the people of the Andes. The first red-skinned, violet-flowering plants reached the Iberian peninsula around 1555. Yellow-skinned varieties reached England and Ireland about 10 years later. But the potato's attraction consisted not in the somewhat unprepossessing tuber, but in the charming flowers as an exotic decoration for the garden. As a food, the potato had rather a negative reputation to begin with. It was only famines that gave the first impetus to potato cultivation. The humble tuber achieved economic significance around the middle of the 18th century. Along with Ireland, Prussia was among the potato pioneers.

> Helps with back pain and strained muscles
> Helps as an additional remedy for lumbago
> Also efficacious for hoof abscesses, colic and equine distemper

Medicinal properties

Freshly prepared, the versatile potato is not only a tasty but also a very healthy food.

An amount of 100 g raw potatoes contains around 78 g water, 15 g carbohydrates, 2.5 g fibre, 2 g protein, organic acids and minerals (potassium, phosphorus, chloride, magnesium etc).

Potatoes are an ideal and healthy food for all, not least because of their alkaline effect on the blood. In naturopathy, potatoes are given against chronic excess acidity. Raw potato juice is recommended for inflammation of the gastric mucous membranes and stomach ulcers. It helps in heartburn, nausea and belching. Due to its diuretic effect, the potato is used to treat oedema.

Eating one kilogram of potatoes without fat and salt every day, improves water retention in the organs and tissues after just a three-day course. The use of potatoes in poultices is especially popular in folk medicine. Warm, moist, potato poultices are suitable wherever warmth is required and at the same time elimination needs to be stimulated. As chest poultices they alleviate coughs and bronchitis and encourage sweating. Potatoes cooked and

A TIP FROM THE VET

Always call the vet urgently in any case of lumbago. The hot poultices are a supplementary measure.

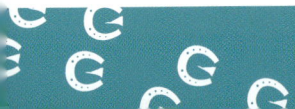

mashed in a towel are also effective for back pain, stiff neck, headaches, bladder infections and osteoarthritis.

Potatoes for horses

Today, the potato no longer plays a big part in horse feeding. Earlier it was given sometimes to work horses as a substitute for grain feed. Cooked potatoes in larger quantities could be added to food.

Hot potato poultices are still a popular remedy for horses. For lumbago, place a bag with cooked and mashed hot potatoes over the region of the back and kidneys, with a woollen blanket on top. Hoof abscesses too, can be treated with a potato poultice.

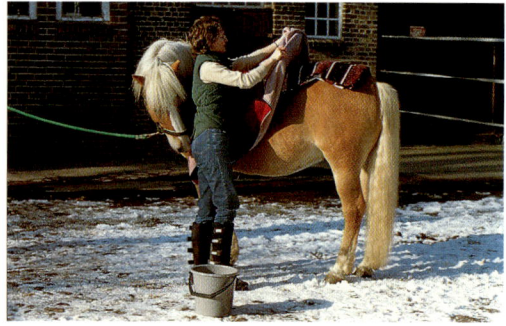 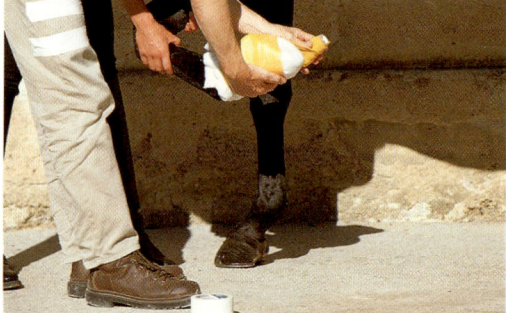

Warm potato poultices are a good supplementary remedy.

IN USE

> USED INTERNALLY

Horses eat potatoes quite happily. Be careful with green and sprouting potatoes, they should never be given to horses.

> USED EXTERNALLY

Hot potato bags as a poultice are a popular remedy for colic and equine distemper also.

Raspberry   *Rubus idaeus*

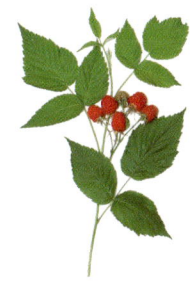

The origins

Findings of raspberry seeds in prehistoric settlements are evidence that raspberries have been used by humans for a very long time. However, raspberry cultivation started only in the Middle Ages. It is not only the tasty fruit, but even more so the blossoms and leaves that find application in naturopathy. Wine, vinegar, syrups and cordials are produced from the sweet fruit. We can enjoy a tasty tea made from the flowers and leaves.

The name 'raspberry' is of uncertain origin, possibly related to 'rough berry'.

Medicinal properties

The pharmaceutical industry utilises raspberries to sweeten children's medicines. But the berries can do much more. They contain tasty ingredients that include citric acid, vitamin C, sugar and mineral salts. Raspberries can be very beneficial both internally and externally. Their refreshing, blood-cleansing and appetite-promoting effects help in rheumatism, angina and various gynaecological conditions. They are used to strengthen the uterus and to encourage milk production. Thanks to their high vitamin C content, raspberries are an effective remedy against scurvy and other vitamin C deficiency disorders. Externally, they help to combat mouth and skin ulcers and inflammation. Even sensitive eyes can be treated with a raspberry infusion.

> Helps mares during foaling
> Acts as a blood-cleanser
> Alleviates rheumatic complaints and is an anti-inflammatory

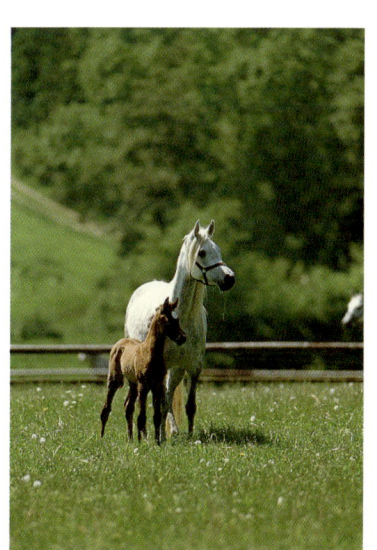

Mares and foals are healthy and spirited.

IN USE

The fruits are popular and a good source of vitamins. They are eaten from the hand as a treat. The leaves, fresh or dried, can be mixed into food.

> DOSAGE

Add 50 g dried leaves or up to 100 g fresh leaves per day to food, or brew into a tea.

> USED INTERNALLY

Even horses find raspberry leaf tea tasty, and it can be poured over food. During flowering, do add a few blossoms since they improve the aroma.

> USED EXTERNALLY

For eye inflammation, use a gauze compress with raspberry leaf tea or decoction. Gauze compresses can be obtained from the pharmacy.

TIP FOR THE RIDER

Riders too, benefit in many ways from raspberry leaf tea rich in vitamin C.

Raspberries for horses

Pregnant mares in particular, can be given raspberry leaves during the last few weeks before foaling and then daily afterwards. This helps to prevent bleeding and strengthens the muscles of the uterus. The afterbirth is expelled more quickly, and the uterus shrinks rapidly.

In older horses who tend to suffer from rheumatism, giving leaves or tea regularly can alleviate the pain. In addition, they benefit from the blood-cleansing effect. Mouth and tooth inflammation can be treated with a tea or decoction, or by simply letting the horse eat the leaves. Eye inflammation too, can be treated with raspberry leaf tea.

Rosehip

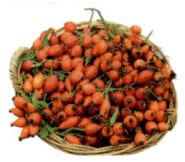

Rosa rugosa / Rosa canina

Dog rose

The origins

The wild rose comes originally from the Mediterranean region. It was taken to America with the Spanish conquerors and established itself in the wild.

In Europe, we find the dog rose almost everywhere, similarly in North Africa and in some parts of Asia. This lovely plant with its pretty blooms prefers open woods, forest margins, copses and sunny hillsides. Its fruit, the rosehips, are used in naturopathy. In earlier times, the wild rose was ascribed healing power against dog bites (rabies), but even without this effect it is a desirable remedy. When harvested in large quantities, the hips have to be extracted arduously with combs from the thorny bushes.

> > Boosts the immune system
> > Strengthens the liver
> > Aids the digestive system

Medicinal properties

The rosehip's high vitamin content is especially well-known. In addition to vitamin C in large amounts (around 5,000 mg per kg) it contains vitamins A and K, niacin, riboflavin and essential oils. Rosehips support treatment for vitamin C deficiency, colds, springtime lethargy and other infections. It is very popular for its flavour and its tolerability when given to children. The Chinese use rosehips as a liver tonic, and they can also be mixed with other 'liver remedies' for detoxification.

A TIP FROM THE VET

In the event of hoof problems and poor hoof growth, give rosehips for a prolonged period.

Rosehip for horses

Rosehips are one of the natural remedies that are easy to procure. Fresh in the autumn, dry for the rest of the year and always as a tea, that is how you should improve your horse's well-being with rosehips. After a long illness and to protect against infections, mix the rosehips with other strength-giving herbs. Since they contain biotin, flavonoids and of course a huge amount of vitamin C, they promote hoof growth, improve the coat and boost the immune system.

We can utilise the liver-fortifying effect in horses suffering from laminitis. Rosehips help to ensure a healthy digestive system, and are beneficial in diarrhoea and constipation.

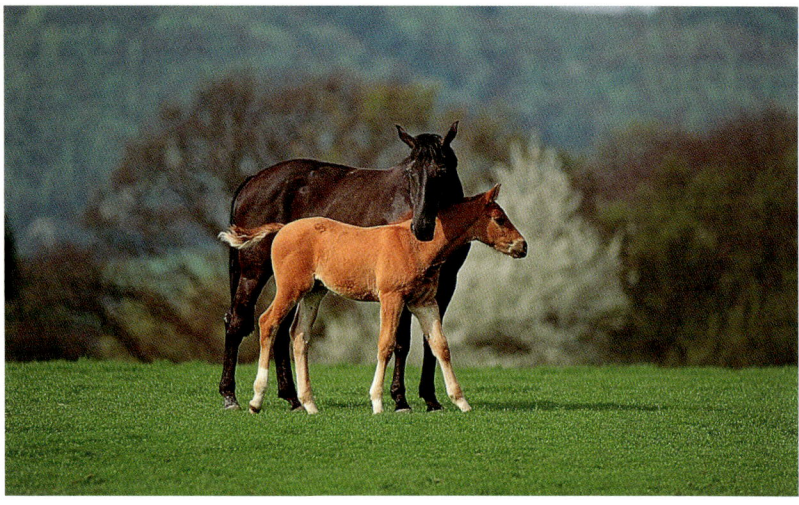

For foaling mares, the vitamin-rich rosehips are a valuable dietary supplement.

IN USE

> USED INTERNALLY

Just like children, horses love rosehip tea. In the autumn, you can mix the freshly-picked small red fruit into food. Dried hips need to be protected from humidity; add them to food every day (chop up just before feeding).

> DOSAGE

You can add 30–40 g of dried fruit to food per day. As a spring course of treatment (change of coat, risk of laminitis, susceptibility to infections), mix rosehip tea with other herbs, for example nettles, green tea and mallow.

Rosemary

Rosemarinus officinalis

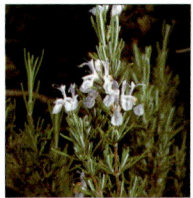

The origins

Queen Isabella of Hungary is supposed to have found relief from her joint pains at the age of 72. This healing was due to an aqueous solution containing lavender, mint and rosemary. We can only guess how much truth there is in this story, but even in antiquity, rosemary was cultivated as a medical herb and a spice. Like many other members of the Labiatae, the mint family, rosemary originated in the Mediterranean region. In the wild, it is found only in warm locations, but it is now cultivated all over the world.

> *> Stimulates the circulation*
> *> Cleanses the blood*
> *> Helps to relieve muscle cramps*

Medicinal properties

The medicinal properties of rosemary are due mainly to its essential oils, including eucalyptol and camphor. It also contains rosmarinic acid and saponins. Internally we value the diuretic, antispasmodic and stimulating effects of rosemary and its positive effect on bile production. Externally, it is wound healing and antiseptic, and used in rheumatism, dental problems and skin complaints. Rosemary additives can be found in many natural remedies for rheumatism, asthma and sprains in the form of ointment, oil or bath salts. When suffering from headaches, instead of immediately swallowing pills it is always worth trying first to rub the forehead with rosemary. During pregnancy, rosemary should be taken in small quantities only.

> **CAUTION**
>
> Rosemary must not be given to pregnant mares. Tournament horses should not be allowed to lick off rosemary oil before an event since camphor comes under anti-doping laws.

Rosemary for horses

Rosemary is a blood-cleansing remedy and has a positive effect on the gastrointestinal system. It stimulates the circulation and helps horses suffering from muscle cramps, stress and nervous restlessness. Together with other herbs, for example verbena and dandelion, it can be used to help with liver problems. Externally, rosemary is invigorating and muscle-relaxing and can be beneficial for small wounds and inflammations.

IN USE

If you grow rosemary in your garden, greenhouse or on the windowsill, you can collect the leaves all year round. Rosemary leaves can be fed to horses fresh or dried. It is available fresh on the market or from your greengrocer.

> DOSAGE

Give a handful of fresh or 15 g dried leaves.

> USED INTERNALLY

For gastrointestinal disorders, prepare an infusion, perhaps in combination with fennel, anise or caraway.

> USED EXTERNALLY

You can also massage with rosemary oil against rheumatism und muscle cramps.

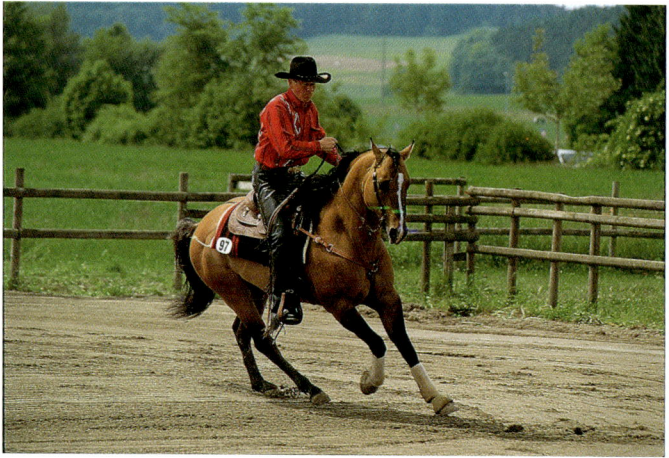

Tournament horses should not be given rosemary before a trial.

Sage

Salvia officinalis

The origins

We can assume that the Romans introduced sage to central and northern Europe, since it originated in the Mediterranean region. By the 9th century it was already common in German monastery gardens. Not only did it heal many disorders, but magical powers were attributed to it. Its many and varied uses range from seasoning dishes to cosmetics to disinfecting linen cupboards. When taken as an infusion, it gets to grips with many an ailment. On dry soils you can plant sage in the garden and use its leaves fresh and dried.

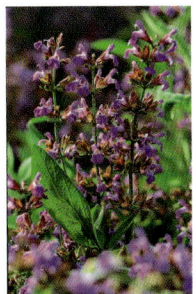

Medicinal properties

The active substances in sage are as varied as its potential uses. The leaves contain essential oils with numerous different chemical structures, saponins, flavonoids and tannins. Sage is antiseptic, antispasmodic, stimulant, carminative, wound-healing and antiperspirant. It promotes bile secretion, regulates menstruation and soothes the digestive organs. Internally and externally, sage relieves many complaints.

> Helps to heal mouth injuries
> Helps in gum inflammation
> Has a positive effect on the digestion
> Natural relief in flu

Sage for horses

For our horses, we value sage especially for treating oral injuries and inflammation. The essential oils in sage have a positive effect on digestion and help to combat flatulence. Sage is a well-known remedy for human and equine flu. It does a good job as a natural antibiotic, even where conventional antibiotics no longer work.

However, both the use of antibiotics and changing to natural remedies should only be done in consultation with the vet and according to the results of a resistance test. Sage is very often an ingredient in cough mixtures, too.

IN USE

Sage is found in almost every cough remedy, also in tinctures for mouth inflammation. In wound ointments for horses too, sage is a well-known additive.

> DOSAGE

Give a handful of fresh or 15 g dried leaves.

> USED INTERNALLY

If you grow sage in your garden, you can feed the leaves to your horse fresh or dried. Sage infusion can be recommended not just for humans: you can also add it to the horse's food.

> USED EXTERNALLY

If your horse has an oral inflammation, you can rinse its mouth with a sage decoction or infusion. A sage–chamomile infusion mixed with honey is equally helpful for disinfecting and a little nicer in flavour.

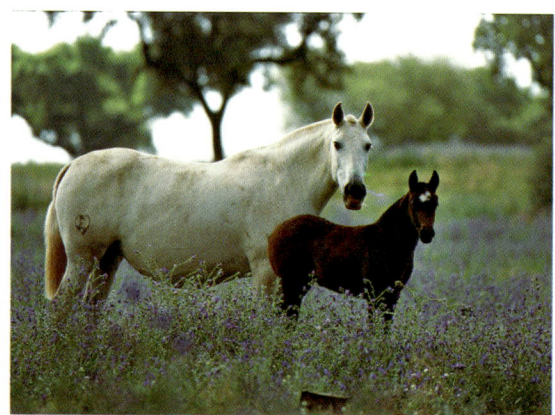

A TIP FROM THE VET

Sage should not be given to pregnant mares. It induces labour and decreases milk production. However, once the foal has been weaned, sage can be beneficial to the mare. Sage is a remedy for acute problems and should not be given over prolonged periods or in excessive doses.

Sage benefits mares only once the foal has been weaned.

Marian thistle
Silybum marianum

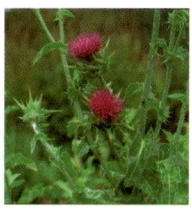

The origins

The Marian thistle's original home was around the Mediterranean and in the Orient. It is now found worldwide.

The Marian thistle is known not only as a medicinal plant, since in earlier times it was also a source of food. A tasty salad can be made from the young leaves. In some countries, the roots and heads are cooked and referred to as wild artichoke. The medicinal effect is ascribed to the leaves, seeds and heads.

> Encourages the activity of the liver
> Protects the liver in severe cases of worms and when taking medications

Medicinal properties

The Marian thistle contains essential oils, histamine, flavonoids and bitter substances. Since it encourages the production of bile, it is valuable for those suffering from liver disorders. Certain substances found in this plant have a beneficial effect in cases of poisoning. Recently it has been discovered that the thistle is efficacious in cardiovascular complaints. Infusions made from the fruits of the Marian thistle are good for the digestion. There are no known side-effects.

CAUTION

The Marian thistle is protected and should not be picked in the wild.

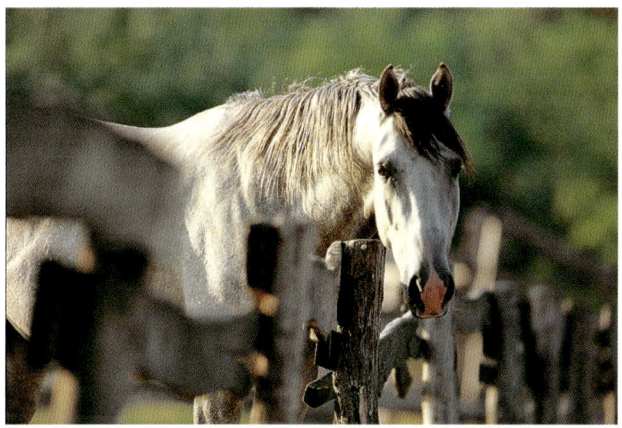

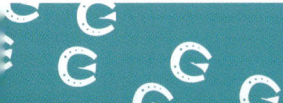

IN USE

Thistles have established themselves on my pasture, and I have discovered that our horses manage them perfectly well and eat them regularly. Our cold blood Alma in particular, seems to regard them as a treat. Perhaps she needs thistles for some condition.

> DOSAGE

Add around 15 g fresh thistle seeds to food daily.

> USED INTERNALLY

Thistle seeds are crushed in a coffee grinder and fed to the horse. You can also make an infusion and pour it over food at meal times. A spring cure is highly recommended. Plant thistles in the pasture or in the garden and delight your horses.

Marian thistle for horses

First and foremost, the Marian thistle is a liver remedy for horses also. It encourages the liver to produce more bile and has a protective effect. It has been thoroughly researched in recent years, and its effect in protecting the liver in the event of medication misuse or poisoning has been demonstrated. Trials in ponies and horses who, due to severe worm infestation or medication had suffered liver damage, confirmed the thistle's positive effect. The plant also has significance for mares, since it contains linolenic acid which is important for the production of female hormones.

St. John's wort *Hypericum perforatum*

> For nervous
and restless
horses
> Promotes
wound
healing
> Helps with
rheumatic
complaints

The origins

In antiquity, St. John's wort garlands were draped over the figures of the gods in order to keep evil spirits away.

Many legends report on the power of this herb, which – it is rumoured – wards off black magic, deters the devil and exerts a force over witches.

Paracelsus praised the effect of St. John's wort 450 years ago. It was used to heal wounds and broken bones. Its special action, however, was exhibited in cases of depression and melancholy.

The genuine St. John's wort thrives almost everywhere in Europe, North America and Asia. In our own garden, the plant delights us with its golden yellow blossoms. Around the feast of St. John the Baptist, 24 June, it contains the largest amount of active substances and should be harvested.

Medicinal properties

Today the witches' magic around St. John's wort is a thing of the past. Modern science has studied this herb under the proverbial microscope. It has been discovered that the active substances in the plant intervene directly in signal transmission in the brain, thereby increasing the level of certain messenger substances that affect mood significantly.

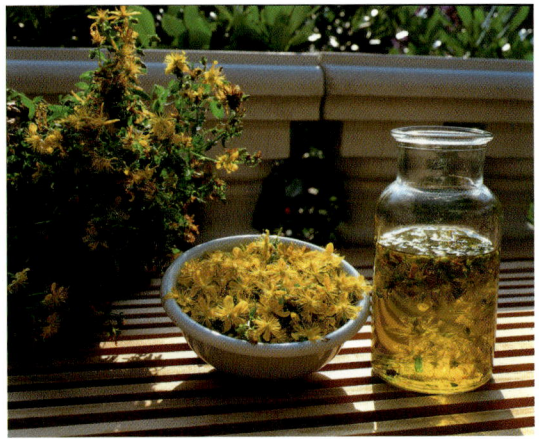

St. John's wort is used in a targeted manner to treat depression, sleep disorders and nervous restlessness. It also acts as an anti-inflammatory, wound-healing, soothing and astringent remedy. In rheumatic pain and burns especially, one feels rapid alleviation of the complaints. St. John's wort is the preferred herbal remedy for nervous disorders.

IN USE

> USED INTERNALLY

When used for calming nerves, it is important to give St. John's wort over a prolonged period. St. John's wort infusion or Hypericum can be effective in homeopathic doses, but always consult your vet.

> USED EXTERNALLY

St. John's wort tincture and St. John's wort oil are available ready-to-use from the pharmacy. For wounds and insect bites, dilute the tincture. St. John's wort oil can be applied undiluted.

You can also prepare a St. John's wort decoction: chop up finely some dried St. John's wort and pour boiling water over it.

A TIP FROM THE VET

St. John's wort contains hypericin, which causes humans and animals to react more sensitively to solar radiation. Therefore, care should be taken in the case of light-sensitive horses who spend all day in the pasture, since taking St. John's wort may lead to sunburn or skin irritations.

St. John's wort for horses

When a horse is unwell or exhibits bad habits, more and more riders consider the possibility of a psychological cause. Poor concentration during a ride, nervousness, anxiety and stress may render contact with horses not only unpleasant but also dangerous. Rider and horse should be relaxed and easy-going with each other when spending time together. Where all the external requirements such as your horse's care, food and exercise are right and it is still jumpy and tense, do try St. John's wort. Not only the horse but also the rider will become calm and relaxed.

Used externally, St. John's wort in the form of oil or tincture promotes wound healing and helps with rheumatic complaints. It should be present in every stable.

Tea tree oil — *Melaleuca alternifolia*

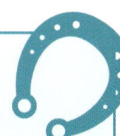

The origins

This wonder tree from Australia and New Zealand has nothing to do with black or green tea. Like eucalyptus, it belongs to the myrtle family and is regarded by the Maoris and the Aborigines, the original inhabitants of New Zealand and Australia, as a healing tree.

James Cook described its healing and revitalising properties, which he tried out on his ship's crew. There is not just one but many species of tea tree, and they differ markedly in their medicinal effects. Their names include tea tree, cajeput, niaouli, manuka and kanuha. I will restrict myself here to the best known species, *Melaleuca alternifolia*, or narrow-leaved tea tree.

> For inhaling against coughs and bronchitis
> Helps against summer eczema, fungal eczema and malanders
> Poultices for pulled muscles and bruises

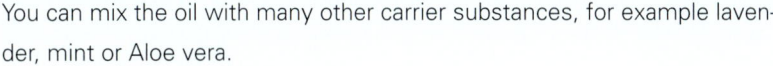

IN USE

You can mix the oil with many other carrier substances, for example lavender, mint or Aloe vera.

> USED EXTERNALLY

Inhalation benefits coughs, bronchitis and respiratory tract disorders. Alternatively, the oil can be applied to the neck, forehead and chest. Apply pure tea tree oil to small wounds, bites, stings or fungal infections. For extensive eczema and other skin and coat problems, mix the oil with carrier substances, or dilute with water and fruit vinegar to make a rinse. You can wash the mane and tail with a tea tree oil shampoo. You can also try tea tree oil with Thuja to treat warts. Mouth rinses with diluted tea tree oil are recommended for inflammation. Even lice are kept away by tea tree oil.

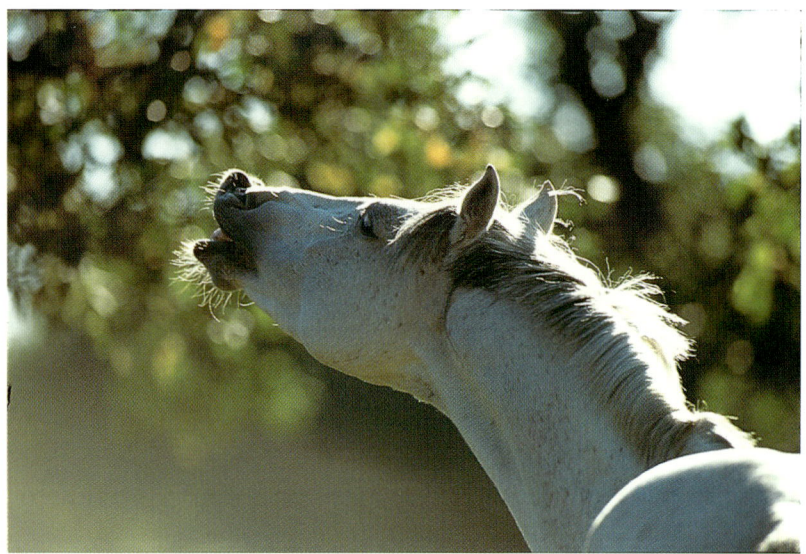

Horses are not keen on the scent of the true tea tree oil.

Medicinal properties

The aborigines used the tea tree for almost all wounds and maladies. They applied its leaves to injuries and used the aroma to treat respiratory complaints. The oil is an exceptionally strong antiseptic and is used against

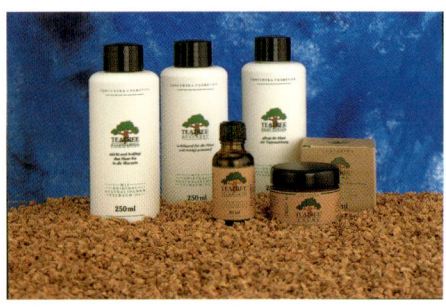

Tea tree products are available for humans and horses.

bacteria, fungi and viruses. It provides valuable first aid for wounds, stings, inflammations, mild burns and acne. Tea tree oil strengthens the immune system and helps to overcome fungal infections, pulled muscles and rheumatism. It can have a beneficial effect on eczema, neurodermatitis and psoriasis. It provides relief for herpes blisters, insect bites and problems involving the lining of the mouth. Tea tree oil is even said to provide help for the soul. It is a fact that the nervous system can be positively influenced via the skin.

Tea tree oil for horses

So how does this wonder remedy help our horses? It certainly cannot replace the vet, but it can bring relief from many minor injuries or support the treatment of more serious complaints. Tea tree oil is efficacious for coughs and bronchitis and stimulates the immune system. It provides quick improvement in cases of thrush, fungal eczema and summer eczema. You can treat malanders and various pests with tea tree oil. As a natural antibiotic, it can be used on its own or to supplement other remedies. In the stable and away, tea tree oil is a reliable method of keeping insects at bay. Poultices with tea tree oil are beneficial for pulled muscles, swellings and rheumatism.

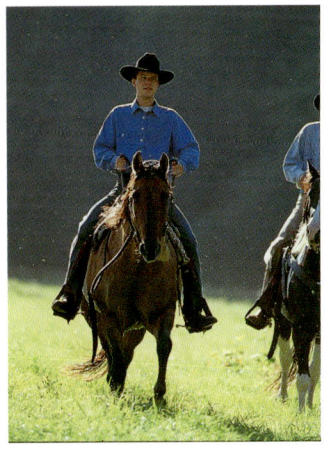

Tea tree oil keeps insects away.

Thyme   *Thymus vulgaris*

> For digestive problems
> Against coughs
> For poorly healing wounds
> Promotes the expulsion of the afterbirth

The origins

The aromatically fragrant thyme prefers dry and sunny locations. It comes originally from the eastern Mediterranean region, but can be found today across the whole of southern Europe, northern and central Asia. In Europe it is cultivated first and foremost as a culinary herb and serves to make numerous medications.

Medicinal properties

Thyme is an ideal natural remedy for coughs and for inflammations of the mucosal membranes and the upper respiratory tract. It is an antiseptic, a good gastric remedy and an antispasmodic, and promotes bile secretion. Externally, it is highly appreciated for its wound-healing, scar-forming properties, especially in poorly healing injuries. As an infusion, thyme is used for bronchitis, coughs, flatulence and stomach cramps. It has proven itself even against stubborn whooping cough.

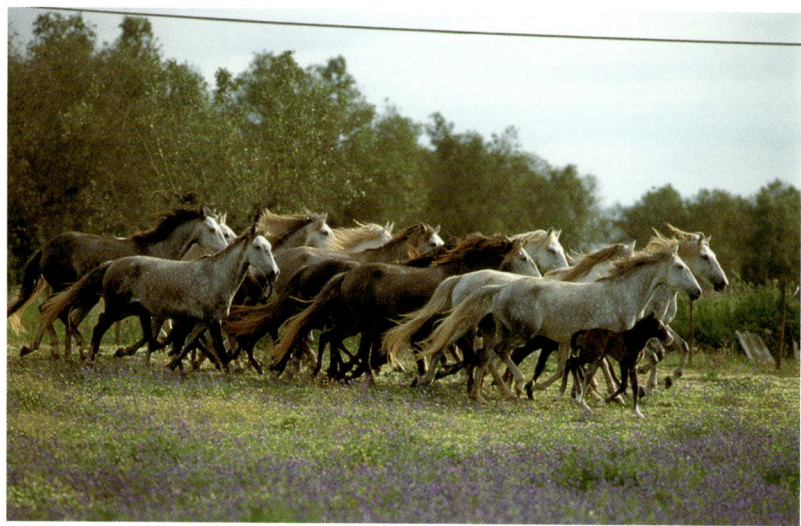

Mares should be given thyme just after foaling.

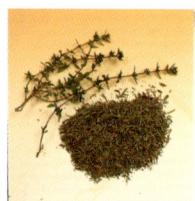

Thyme for horses

Since thyme overcomes flatulence and suppresses fermentation processes, it is given to horses for all digestive problems. If your horses suffer from coughs, bronchitis or inflammation of the respiratory organs, here too you can consider thyme and brew it for them as an infusion. Thyme is also reputed to have an anthelmintic effect, and supports conventional treatments for worms. In mares, thyme promotes the expulsion of the afterbirth and can be beneficial for uterine infections. Poorly healing, purulent wounds and fungal skin problems can be treated with a thyme decoction.

IN USE

Thyme can be used fresh or dried. Fresh thyme is available from the greengrocer, or dried from the pharmacy. Almost all cough products for horses contain thyme, and it can also be found in other veterinary remedies.

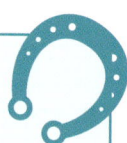

> DOSAGE

Mix a handful of fresh thyme into food as necessary.

> USED INTERNALLY

Horses prefer thyme as an infusion; its fragrant aroma is good for the appetite.

> USED EXTERNALLY

To treat wounds, inflammation or fungal infections, brew an infusion and wash the affected area carefully.

Valerian   *Valeriana officinalis*

All-heal

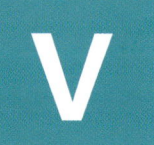

The origins

An Egyptian physician mentioned valerian in the 9th century. In the Middle Ages it was even regarded as a cure-all. Sometimes it was used as a febrifuge. Today, valerian is considered one of the best tranquillisers for nervous disorders.

The native population of Mexico took a particular kind of valerian against tiredness, and to help them endure privations.

The peculiarly unpleasant odour of valerian has a strong attraction for cats.

Valerian grows in both humid and dry locations in woods, copses and ditches.

> For soothing nervous over-excitation
> Boosts the immune system
> For cramp colic
> For muscle relaxation

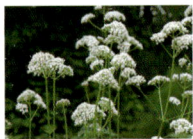

Medicinal properties

Valerian has, first and foremost, a wonderfully calming effect without being habit-forming. In some cases it is also used as an appetite suppressant.

Valerian can provide relief in disorders of the gastrointestinal tract and get rid of flatulence and cramps. It has a balancing and regulating effect on the autonomic nervous system. It is a true and yet completely harmless remedy for stress, with whose help one can better endure hectic and restless times. At the same time, it is the remedy of choice for insomnia resulting from nervous exhaustion, disturbing thoughts or excessive mental activity.

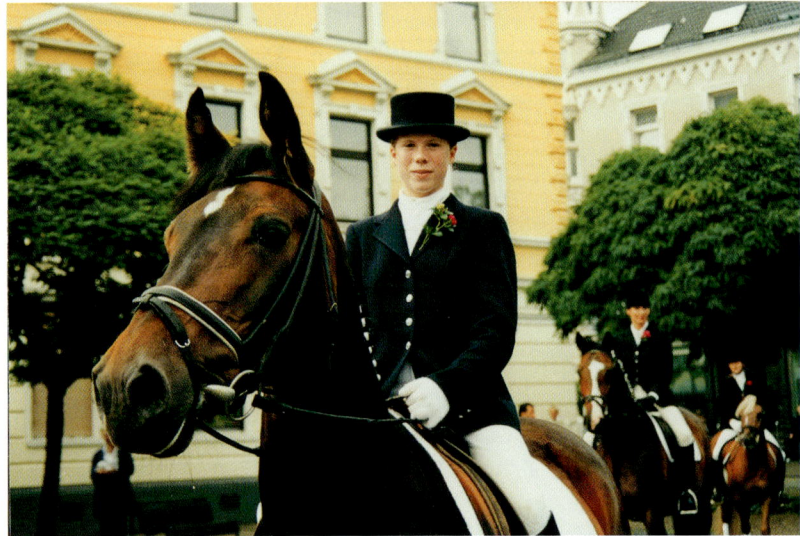

Nervous before the tournament? Valerian soothes both horse and rider.

Valerian for horses

A TIP FROM THE VET

Even with the same dose, valerian can affect each horse differently.

The calming effect of valerian is manifested in full in horses, too. It relaxes hectic and anxious horses without impairing their performance.

Horses that react with cramp colic to every change in their environment, can be soothed with valerian. Stress resulting from tournaments or a change of stabling, owner or carer can be staved off with valerian.

Even bad habits caused by nervous over-stimulation can often be corrected with this healing herb.

Valerian is also said to have an anthelmintic effect in horses. However, it is no substitute for proper worming.

Externally, valerian is recommended for wound healing and for muscle relaxation.

IN USE

> USED INTERNALLY

Valerian can be mixed with food as a crushed and ground root (around 15 g daily). As a liquid product, it is given as drops drizzled onto bread or sugar or sprayed with a syringe (without a needle) into the mouth.

When mixed with fruit vinegar, the somewhat peculiar valerian odour is no longer noticed by the horse.

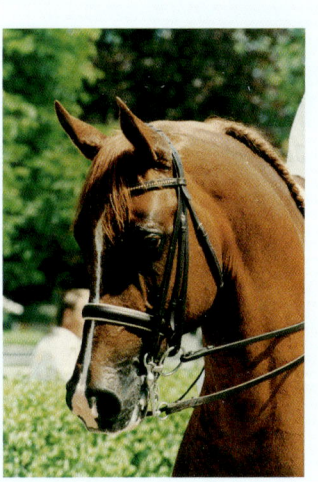

> USED EXTERNALLY

Place a sterile gauze swab soaked in valerian on the affected area, or massage the mixed liquid into the strained muscle region.

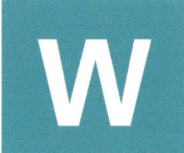

Water

The origins

The use of water in the healing arts has been known since antiquity.

Treatment with water, also known as hydrotherapy, offers a plethora of therapeutic options.

Medicinal properties

Among the best known therapeutic applications of water are those developed by the German priest, Sebastian Kneipp. The term 'gush' was also coined for these methods by Kneipp. It would take far more than we have space for in this book to explain all of Kneipp's techniques: this would require intensive study and practice. Hydrotherapy activates respiration and metabolism and the lymph and immune systems, and via the nervous

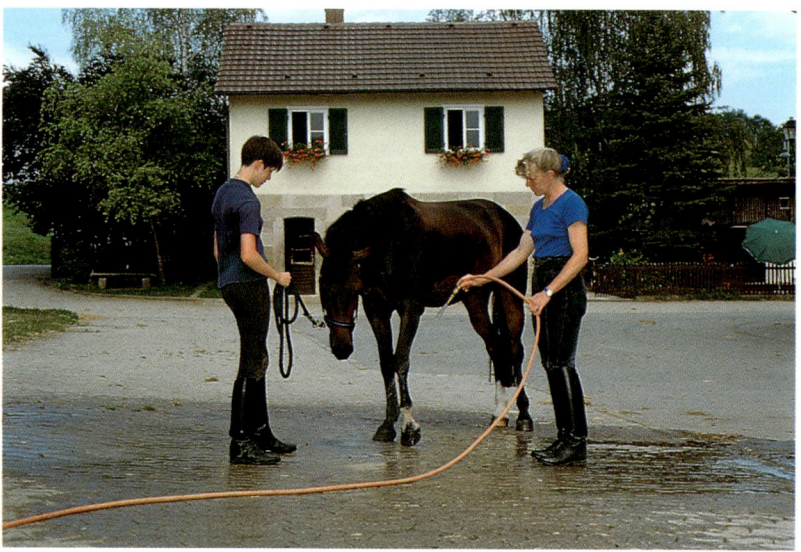

It's always good to be refreshed in the summer.

pathways to the skin also stimulates the internal organs. With the help of water, the body can regulate its heat balance and react to changes in temperature.

Water for horses

In the summer particularly, after an outing, most horses like to be refreshed with a water hose. But before you get going, note the following points:

1. Direct cold water only at warm parts of the body.
2. Do not direct on a full stomach.
3. Do not direct on a completely empty stomach (give the horse something to eat about half an hour beforehand).
4. No water therapy in the presence of total exhaustion or fever.
5. Do not hose horses with water in a draughty place. Their legs are very sensitive and susceptible to illness.

Intensive training under a rider, long trail rides and frequent tournament sports, especially show jumping and riding on heavy soil, can all expose the legs to very high stress. Over-exertion, pulled muscles, bruises and other minor injuries can be treated with gushes of water.

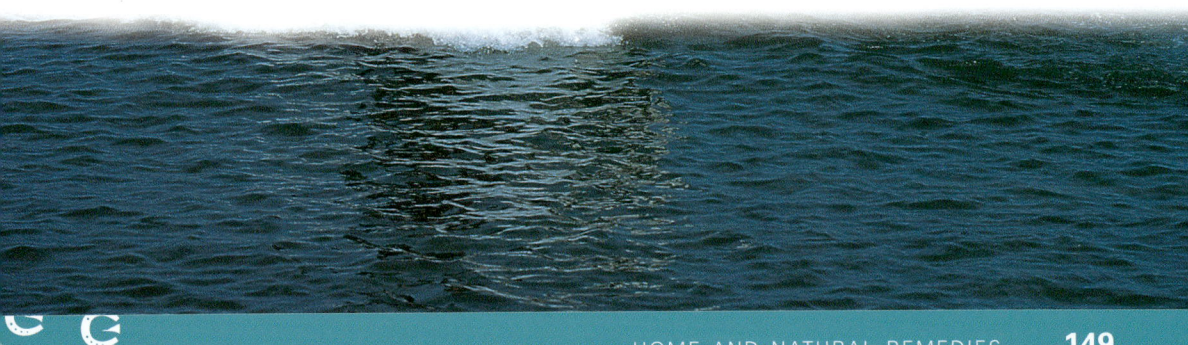

IN USE

Over-exerted and swollen legs can be cooled down with a water hose. Move the hose slowly from bottom to top. Do not keep it aimed for too long at one spot, which could get too cold. Use every opportunity to walk with your horse through water or stand in it. Once they have become familiar with it, most horses like going into water. They drink from the stream or strike playfully with their front legs. Experienced horsepeople swear even today by the healing powers of a cold, rapidly flowing brook.

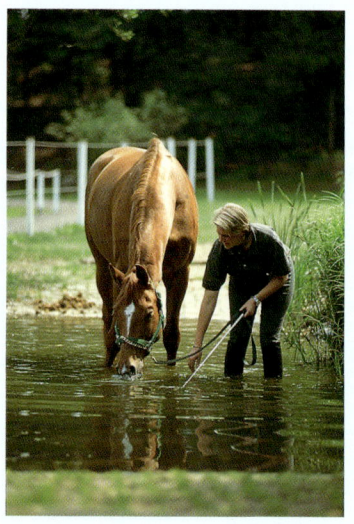

If you have nothing else available, a bucketful of water will work also. You can add to the water various supplements, for example basic aluminium acetate, arnica tincture or cider vinegar. You need a little patience for water therapy, but it's worth your while. My mare Kaitra suffers from laminitis and early every morning she was led slowly through tall wet grass. Often this was arduous and she didn't want to go, but after 30 minutes she could walk better again. At noon she was allowed to stand for 20 minutes in a bucket of water with basic aluminium acetate. Nux vomica D6 and Ginkgo biloba were given internally.

> Helps to treat wounds and burns
> Good for tendon problems
> Benefits rheumatism and arthritis

White cabbage — *Brassica oleracea*

The origins

Opinion is divided when it comes to the image of cabbage. From time immemorial it has been known and celebrated as a star among the medicinally beneficial vegetables, but for long has been regarded in the kitchen as 'poor people's food'. In the years following WWII it was frowned upon, as was everything that constantly went on the table in times of hunger.

Today, cabbage has become socially respectable again throughout the world, and is regarded as a very healthy delicacy whether raw or cooked.

Medicinal properties

Nutritionists are unanimous: eat a portion of cabbage several times a week, or better still every day. In addition to vitamin C and B2, white cabbage contains vitamin B12, minerals, iron, potassium, calcium and lactic acid bacteria, especially when prepared as sauerkraut. Cabbage is regarded as an 'anti-cancer remedy' and fights bacteria. It is an ideal food when suffering from gastrointestinal problems, it strengthens the immune system and stimulates the digestion. Cabbage is said to lower blood sugar levels. In addition, it is ideal when dieting and for high blood pressure. It is low-calorie, filling food.

IN USE

> USED EXTERNALLY

For all the complaints listed above, make a cabbage compress. The greenest, thickest leaves are highest in active substances. The leaves are washed and the stalk ends removed. Crush them with a rolling pin or a bottle until soft. Then arrange them criss-cross in layers and attach them carefully with a bandage. After six to eight hours remove the poultice, and repeat with new leaves if needed. This is a cheap but very effective treatment. It helps the rider just as much as the horse!

White cabbage for horses

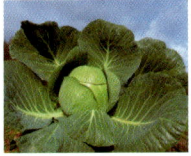

Internally, give horses no more than two or three leaves to eat, otherwise there is a risk of colic. Should your horse end up in a white cabbage field and

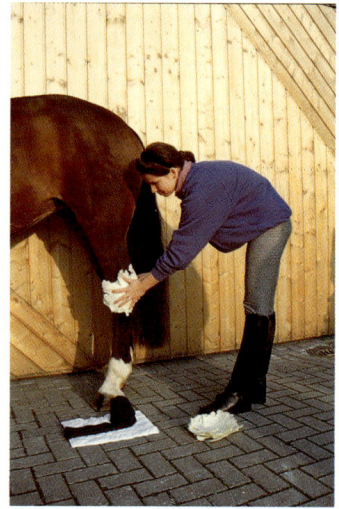 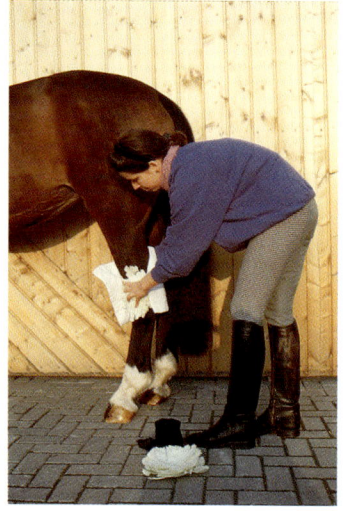 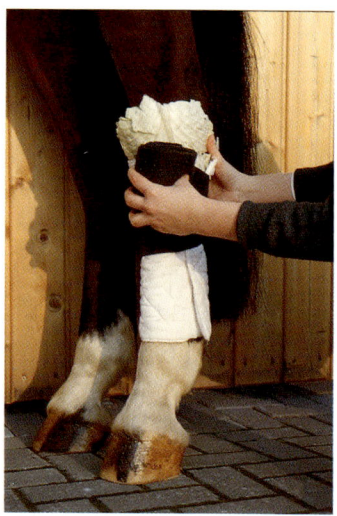

The cabbage poultice . . .   *is fixed in place with a cloth . . .*   *and a bandage.*

consume a lot, call the vet at once. Externally, however, white cabbage is an invaluable remedy for many ailments. Place cabbage on inflammations of all kinds and anywhere: wounds, ulcers, minor burns, contusions, swellings, rheumatism, arthritis and other complaints, especially chronic ones, also old and poorly healing wounds. In horses with tendon problems, it is always possible to try a cabbage poultice in addition to veterinary procedures.

> Analgesic, dehydrating effect
> Helps to deal with rheumatism and exhaustion
> Can be given over a prolonged period

Willow bark   *Salicaceae*

Salix alba – white willow

The origins

The white willow and other willow species were recognised as medicinal plants from early on. The clay tablets of the Assyrians and Babylonians mention medicines made from willow blossoms. The use of remedies prepared from parts of the willow is described in writings from ancient Egypt (1551–1070 BC). They utilised willow leaves, twigs and bark against painful wounds and inflammation. Hippocrates (460–377 BC) prescribed a willow bark infusion against joint inflammation, pain and fever. A prescription exists in which willow bark ashes mixed with parsley are recommended as a remedy for coughs in mules and horses. The ashes mixed with water were also used against equine mange. Hildegard of Bingen recommended the willow for pain and fever. In mythology, willows are described as witches' trees. And if someone suffering from toothache visits a willow, the complaint is supposed to disappear. Traditionally, proximity to a willow helps in cases of gout, rheumatism and menstrual complaints.

Medicinal properties

Investigations of the willow bark gave rise to the world's best-known analgesic: aspirin. Researchers made a discovery in 1828, from which aspirin was later developed. The active agent in aspirin, acetylsalicylic acid, came originally from willow bark. However, other valuable substances such as flavonoids, and tannins are found in the willow. A number of possible uses are described in naturopathy. New studies even promise benefits in diabetes mellitus.

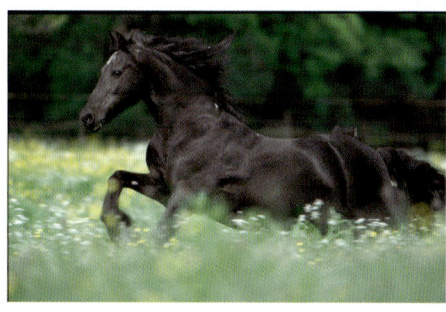

Joy in movement is important to every horse.

Willow bark for horses

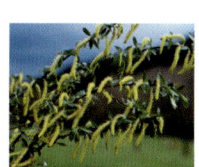

Have you ever placed willow twigs in your horse's or pony's pasture or stable? You will discover that all equines gnaw at the bark enthusiastically. Most animals know what's good for them. This is the easiest way to use willow bark. The leaves are also taken readily, and their effect is similar to that of the bark.

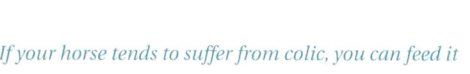

If your horse tends to suffer from colic, you can feed it fresh willow leaves.

Willow is recommended in particular for treating rheumatism, inflammation, fever and a tendency to suffer from colic and cramps. Compared with synthetic salicin compounds, the willow has the advantage of not giving rise to side-effects. It can be given over prolonged periods and is easy to obtain. Willows grow everywhere in northern temperate regions. They like moist soils, rivers and streams.

IN USE

> USED INTERNALLY

The best harvesting time is spring. Fresh leaves can then be fed daily, two to three handfuls. With the bark, it is recommended to decoct 30 g in one litre of water and feed around 140 ml per day. The obtained decoction is best given directly into the mouth with a syringe. This method has proved more effective than simply distributing the fluid over food.

> USED EXTERNALLY

Stressed muscle groups can be massaged with the decoction after a tough ride. Especially in winter, when horses can get bored in the pasture or the stable, they are glad of the chance to nibble on a couple of willow branches and twigs.

> For sprains and contusions
> Against muscle stiffness
> For eye inflammation

Witch hazel   *Hamamelis virginiana*

The origins

Witch hazel was one of the most important remedies of the Native Americans. Its healing powers in man and beast were greatly valued, and utilised for many ailments. Witch hazel occurs mainly in the humid forests of North America and especially Canada. Its bark, twigs and leaves are used in naturopathy.

Medicinal properties

As modern enlightened people, we no longer believe in the miraculous powers that Native Americans used to attribute to the witch hazel. But even without magic, this shrub is a useful medicinal plant. The witch hazel's leaves and bark contain a very special tannin, gallic acid. It has an astringent and vasoconstrictive effect. Numerous ointments, tinctures and lotions contain Hamamelis water. It helps with skin problems, varicose veins and haemorrhoids, and for a long time has been an established ingredient in cosmetic products.

TIP FOR THE RIDER

Witch hazel benefits both the rider and the horse when suffering from stiff muscles and tired legs, but also helps to staunch bleeding from open wounds.

IN USE

> USED EXTERNALLY

Hamamelis products are available commercially in a variety of forms, also mixed with other herbs, for example arnica. An ointment can act as first aid for many small wounds. You can also buy Hamamelis leaves and prepare a decoction yourself. Pour water over the leaves (1 cup of water for 1 tablespoon of leaves), boil up briefly, then brew for 15 minutes and use the decoction either warm, e.g. for the eyes, or cold for pulled muscles.

Witch hazel for horses

In horses, witch hazel is used mainly externally. It is of great benefit in treating sprains and contusions. After a strenuous ride or hard training, it refreshes aching muscles and tired legs. Ulcers, wounds, saddle sores and

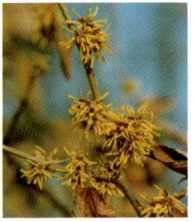

bruises are alleviated with witch hazel. The boiled decoction is good in compresses for inflamed eyes, often caused by a windy day on the pasture. Witch hazel is especially recommended in combination with eyebright. The use of arnica and witch hazel can also help with bruised soles. Bleeding can be stopped more quickly thanks to the witch hazel's astringent property.

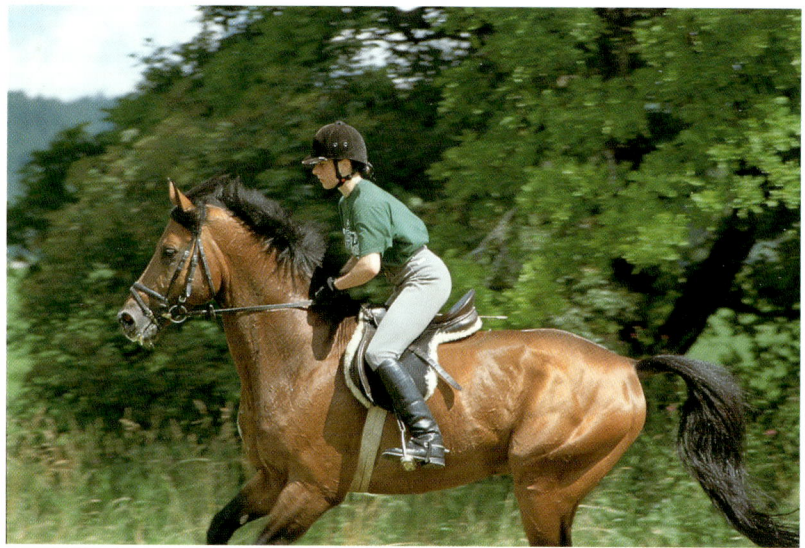

Witch hazel is good after a long, strenuous ride.

Y

Yarrow

Achillea millefolium

The origins

> Combats flies
> Good for laminitis and navicular disease
> First aid for bleeding

The healing powers of this plant were discovered very early on. On the Feast of the Assumption, it was bound into bunches and consecrated. Yarrow is used as a remedy for numerous complaints. It occurs in meadows, pasture and by the side of roads nearly everywhere in Europe.

The ancient Greek hero, Achilles, is said to have treated the wounds of his soldiers with yarrow, which gave rise to the plant's Latin name.

Medicinal properties

Once again, it is the essential oils that are responsible for much of the yarrow's useful effects. To this we can add resins, tannins, organic acids, phosphorus, potassium and an alkaloid. Its many medicinal properties have made it a popular folk remedy. Yarrow has an antiseptic, astringent, haemostatic, antispasmodic and wound-healing effect. The parts used are the leaves, fruits and the tips of the blossoms. It helps in acne, haemorrhoids, varicose veins and wounds. Dandruff and dull hair can also be treated effectively with yarrow.

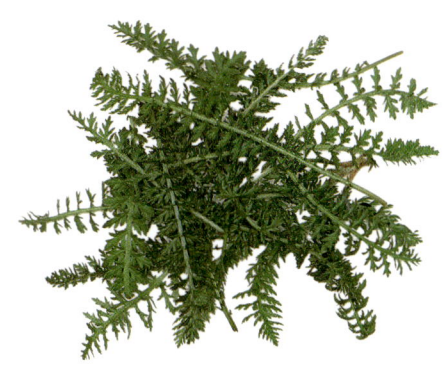

Yarrow is often regarded as a female remedy. It is beneficial in menstrual complaints involving cramp-like pain.

It is a popular ingredient of blood-cleansing infusions for spring and autumn cures. In earlier times, yarrow was used in beer brewing instead of hops.

Yarrow for horses

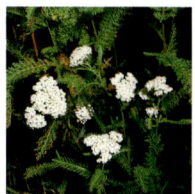

When hanging up garlic in the stable, you can add a bunch of yarrow in order to keep flies away.

Horses can be rubbed vigorously with yarrow to protect them against flies. Given internally, yarrow is good for bladder infections and rheumatism. It stimulates the appetite and can even be given to feverish horses. Yarrow improves the circulation in the upper blood vessels and can be given for laminitis and navicular disease. Applied externally, yarrow is a first-aid remedy for bleeding, for example nosebleeds and wounds.

IN USE

Yarrow is still found today in almost every pasture. Horses like eating it, and it does them the most good when taken internally. If there is enough yarrow growing in your pasture, you can simply dry bunches of it. You can use the plant for inhalation to treat a cough. In case of a fresh wound, simply place yarrow leaves on it as first aid until the vet arrives. For horses you can also use yarrow oil. It has a soothing, analgesic and anti-inflammatory effect on skin complaints. Yarrow is available in dried form and is an ingredient in many herbal mixtures for horses.

> DOSAGE

Feed around 30 g dried yarrow daily or pour the infusion over food.

> USED INTERNALLY

Add a herbal mixture or infusion to food.

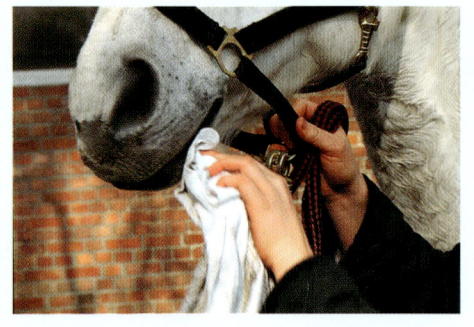

> USED EXTERNALLY

Wounds are treated with fresh leaves or compresses with the infusion. For horses you can also use yarrow oil.

> Ensures
a balanced
intestine
> Ensures
healthy
intestinal flora
after giving
antibiotics
> Good for
older horses

Yoghurt and whey

Medicinal properties

Problems of the abdomen and stomach, of the intestines and digestion, are as common as they are annoying and disagreeable. Some foods contain useful bacteria that benefit the digestive organs and the entire immune system.

Sauerkraut, yoghurt, kefir and soured milk are teeming with bacteria that unleash their valuable effect in the gut. Anyone can ingest lactic acid bacteria very easily by eating whey or yoghurt. It is important to use live culture yoghurt, which can even be made at home.

IN USE

> DOSAGE

If your horse is not keen on yoghurt, it can be added to food with the familiar infusion or honey. Even my elderly horses, who can no longer eat so well and prefer to drool over mash, are given a daily portion of yoghurt with bananas and honey, mixed into their food. Bran is also suitable, mixed with warm water and yoghurt. You may give around 200–250 ml of yoghurt twice a day.

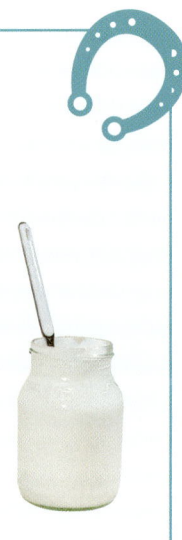

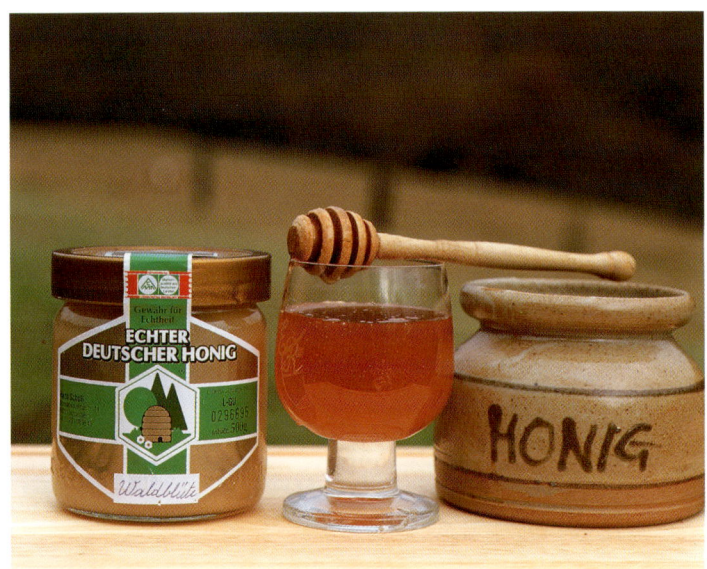

Older horses remain fit with yoghurt, honey and herbal tea.

Yoghurt for horses

For years, I believed that milk and milk products do not necessarily have a place on a horse's menu, however in an effort to help our old horses with somewhat damaged teeth in winter, it was decided to try yoghurt in addition to mash, bran, bananas, linseed oil, beetroot, numerous herbs, infusions and vitamins. A pot of yoghurt was added to Polly's usual food mixture. She announced her approval with a loud lip-smacking noise. Now, she also eats yoghurt on its own. Do experiment to find out what your horse likes.

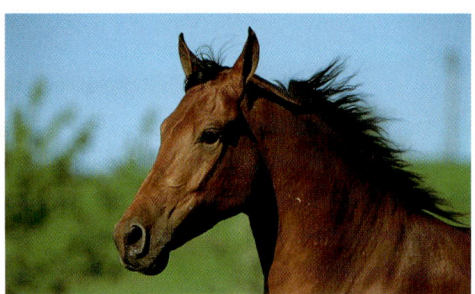

Yoghurt is popular with horses also.

Unfortunately, our horses' intestinal balance is not always as it should be. Antibiotics need to be used in certain medical conditions in order to prevent harm to our horses' health or even save their lives. Antibiotics destroy the natural flora in the gut. Here the rider can aid the horse responsibly. 'Live' yoghurt helps, and horses are happy to eat it.

A varied diet

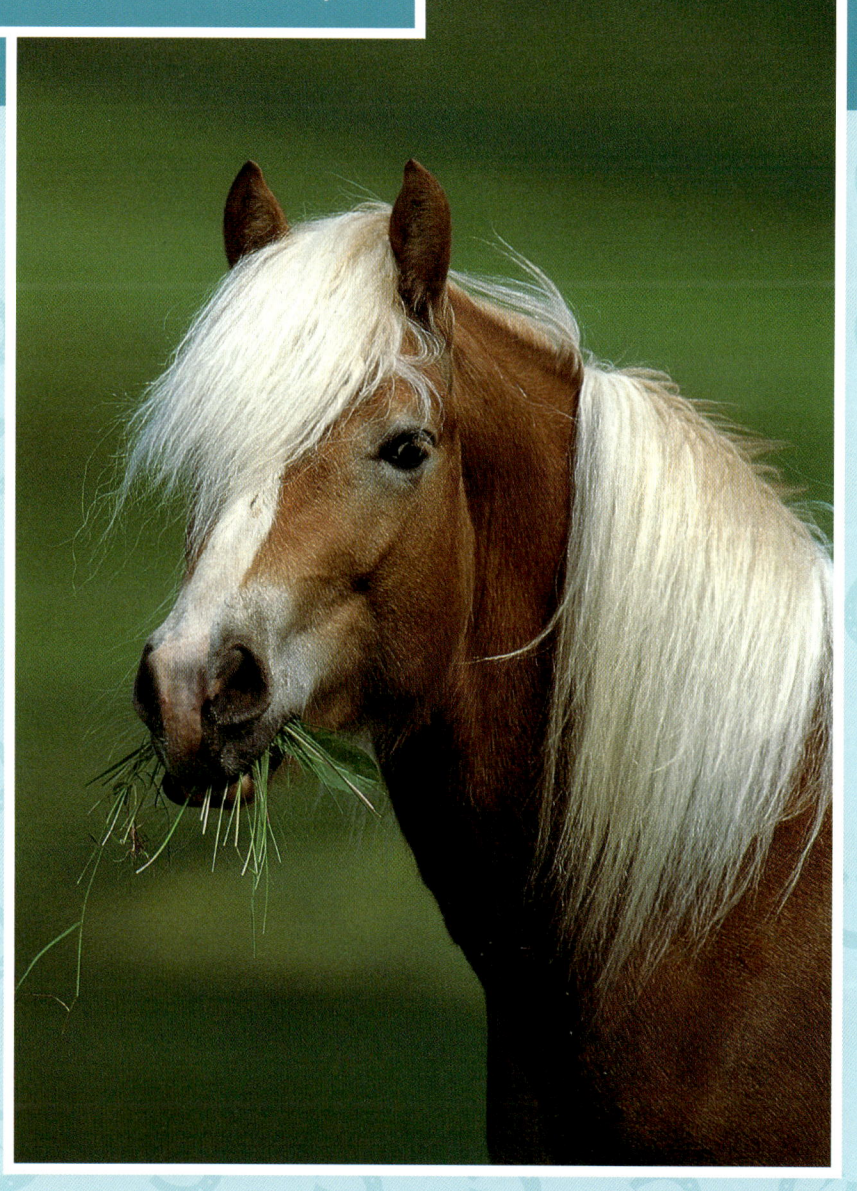

Fruit for horses

As we know, our horses have a sweet tooth. According to the old saying, you can get your way with a sugar cube and a whip, although we should update it and omit the whip. However, sugar too is not a good solution for rewarding horses. The dressage rider's trick of giving the occasional sugar cube before work in order to stimulate the mouth's activity is fine. As a daily treat, however, there are healthier alternatives.

Apples and **pears** are well-known and greatly valued in horse circles. They are quite safe to give in large quantities. In addition, whichever is your favourite fruit, see whether your horse might perhaps be equally keen on it.

In winter, **oranges** and **tangerines** are a very balanced source of vitamin C. Before your stable is overrun with coughing, give the horses one or two oranges a day; they are a good preventive and support any treatment.

In the case of nervous and elderly horses in particular, don't forget **bananas**. Lovely soft bananas are an excellent source of magnesium and also a delicacy. Both horse and rider see many things more philosophically when they eat bananas regularly. I always have the impression that the older horses are disappointed if I enter the stable without bananas. As far as our goat Rosi is concerned, I must hide the bananas quickly otherwise she'll snap them all up and gobble them complete with skin. Your greengrocer is sure to give you his squishy fruits once he knows who they are intended for.

When out on a walk or ride, pick some **rosehips** for your horse. They enrich the wintertime diet. Rosehips have a high vitamin C, E and K content, and promote a healthy digestive system.

Like so much else, I learned from our pony Polly that horses love **raspberries** just as much as people do. Years ago, I had a small raspberry hedge in the garden. When Polly stayed, her first visit was always to the hedge to eat the raspberries. This is also how I discovered her fondness for parsley and chives.

With exotic fruits too, you can think of your horses. One or two peeled **kiwis** a day can be added to the food. Once horses learn to know them, they will eat all fruits as treats from your hand.

Pasture with fruit trees

An orchard pasture offers a wonderful change for horses, but you need to get them accustomed to it slowly. You cannot take a horse used to being stabled and then suddenly in late summer or autumn let it graze for hours in an orchard meadow, since colic would then be pre-programmed.

You should be especially careful in pastures with plum trees. Some horses eat plums whole with the stones and can suffer from poisoning, which may even be fatal.

Our ponies have developed an amazing technique for spitting out the stones. Plum stones contain prussic acid, which in large amounts is toxic. If you give your horse plums, you must always remove the stones.

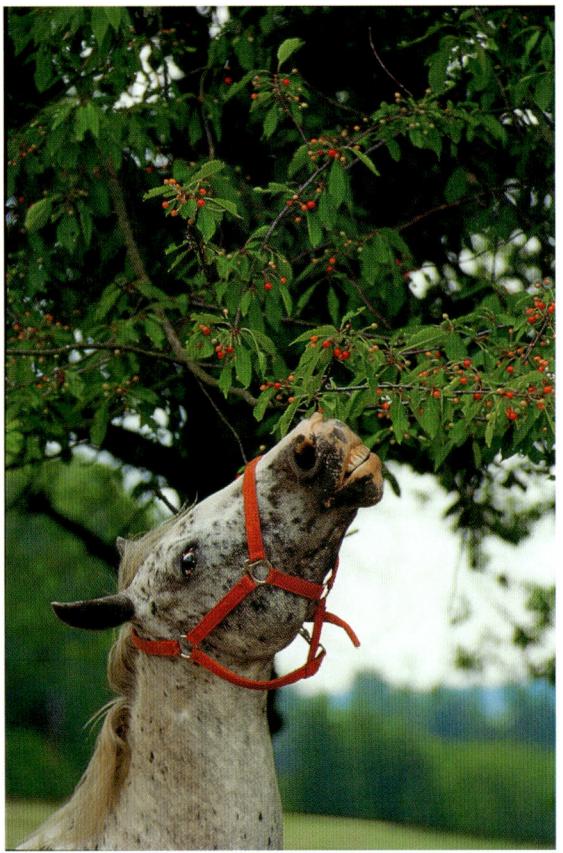

Cherries from the neighbour's garden? But please, without stones . . .

Teatime in the stable

All horses like infusions and drink them with relish. Some prefer them as a supplement to their drinking water, but the majority are happy to drink them on their own. The most popular method is to pour the infusion over food or mix it into the food.

Especially during the cold season, you should offer your horse a lukewarm infusion. Infusions are an ideal source of vitamins, stimulate the metabolism and have a fortifying and healing effect on numerous health disorders.

Since every horse has its favourite infusion, do you know which one your horse prefers? This is one way to make food supplements, for example cough medicine, more palatable. If your horse is not interested in eating, you can persuade it to take food by adding a tasty infusion.

Infusion recipes

Find out your horse's favourite infusion and mix in various supplements. It is fun to try various alternatives and accumulate personal experience. Develop your own ideas, and see what goes well together and what benefits your horse. Combine no more than five different herbs. For an infusion recipe you need only around 100 g fresh or 30–50 g dried herbs. Pour about 500 ml boiling water on the herbs (except green tea) and let the infusion brew for 10 to 15 minutes. Let it cool down to a lukewarm temperature, and give the infusion together with the herbs. If

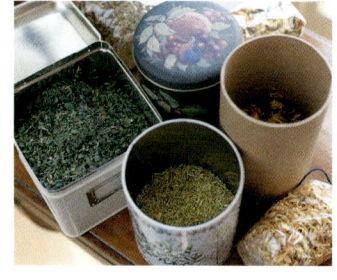

you have no herbs available, you can also use teabags. The best and most effective method is to brew a fresh infusion each time. If this is impossible, you can keep it warm in a Thermos flask for several hours. In the event of gastrointestinal disorders and coughs, the infusion should be given lukewarm. All infusions can be enriched and improved with honey, grape sugar or other vitamin sources.

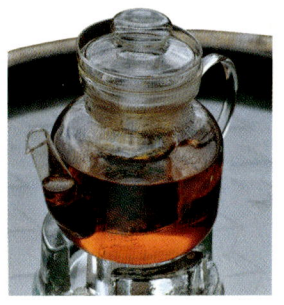

Tasty favourites

Fennel, caraway, anise.

Cough infusion

Anise, fennel, liquorice, thyme, yarrow, horsetail, spruce needles, coltsfoot, chamomile, sage, marsh mallow root, Iceland moss, mallow, buckhorn, garlic, oregano, comfrey, coneflower, rosehip.

My tried and tested mixture

Thyme, coltsfoot, sage.

Circulation tea for elderly horses

Garlic, mistletoe, hawthorn, nettle, anise, fennel, caraway, ginseng, coneflower, hay flowers, green tea, peppermint, dandelion.

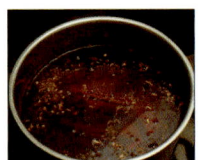

My tried and tested mixture

Green tea, mistletoe, hawthorn.

Fitness infusion to fortify the immune system

Nettle, marigold, coneflower, ginseng, green tea, garlic, goosegrass, rosemary, rosehip, Iceland moss.

My tried and tested mixture

Coneflower, rosehip, ginseng.

Gastrointestinal infusion

Anise, fennel, caraway, chamomile, peppermint, comfrey, marsh mallow, liquorice, valerian, elm, meadowsweet, fenugreek.

My tried and tested mixture

Anise, fennel, caraway.

Calming infusion for nervous horses

Lavender, valerian, St. John's wort, chamomile, lime blossom, hops, magnesium.

My tried and tested mixture

Lavender, hops, valerian.

Skin and coat infusion for eczema

Nettle, horsetail, walnut leaves, rosehip, burdock root, chamomile, marigold, garlic, coneflower, goosegrass, meadowsweet, dandelion.

My tried and tested mixture

Nettle, Iceland moss, burdock root.

Circulation tea for laminitis

Nettle, dandelion, garlic, comfrey, goosegrass, burdock, Marian thistle, hawthorn.

My tried and tested mixture

Nettle, dandelion, comfrey.

Rheumatism/osteoarthritis infusion

Willow bark, hay flowers, heartsease, nettle, garlic, green tea, goosegrass, meadowsweet, marigold, devil's claw, fruit vinegar, rosemary, buckwheat, hawthorn, dandelion, algae.

My tried and tested mixture

Nettle, meadowsweet, goosegrass, chamomile.

Blood-cleansing infusion

Nettle, garlic, goosegrass, birch leaves, dandelion, walnut leaves, horsetail, heartsease.

My tried and tested mixture

Nettle, dandelion.

Stabilising tea for hormone disorders

Monk's pepper, raspberries, ginseng.

Plant oils for more vitality

Oils are a popular food supplement for horses. We should not forget, however, that horses cannot digest large quantities of oils. When used in appropriate doses, they can make a positive contribution to maintaining good health. It is important to make sure that the oils have been cold pressed and are 100% natural.

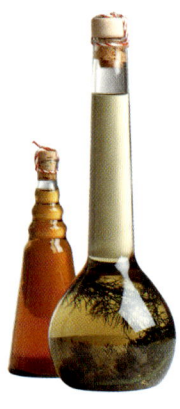

Plant oils contain polyunsaturated fatty acids, which enhance performance. Ideally, they are used to benefit ill and weak horses and those suffering from diet-related deficiencies. Vitality is increased, the muscles strengthened, and coat and skin problems positively influenced. In foals, weight increase during the growth phase is promoted.

Plant oils have a high vitamin content, especially vitamins A, E and B. Vitamin E stimulates the regeneration of all organs and protects against harmful environmental effects. Vitamin A is important for the skin, coat and eyes. Vitamin B fortifies the nerves and also has a positive effect on the hooves, coat and skin.

Possible oils for horses include:

1.   Linseed oil
2.   Sunflower oil
3.   Thistle oil
4.   Olive oil in small quantities.

Remember that oils should be given only in small amounts, divided equally between all the meals. It's best to drizzle a tablespoon of oil over the food three times a day, at each mealtime. Never give a larger amount just once a day. Horses have no gall bladder and cannot utilise large quantities of fats.

Caution: horses suffering from laminitis are better off without oil. Those that do little work, eat all day long and are healthy and round, need no oil. Providing oil makes sense in the case of weak, elderly horses and those subjected to maximum demands such as trail rides, endurance riding, tournaments or other unusual exertions.

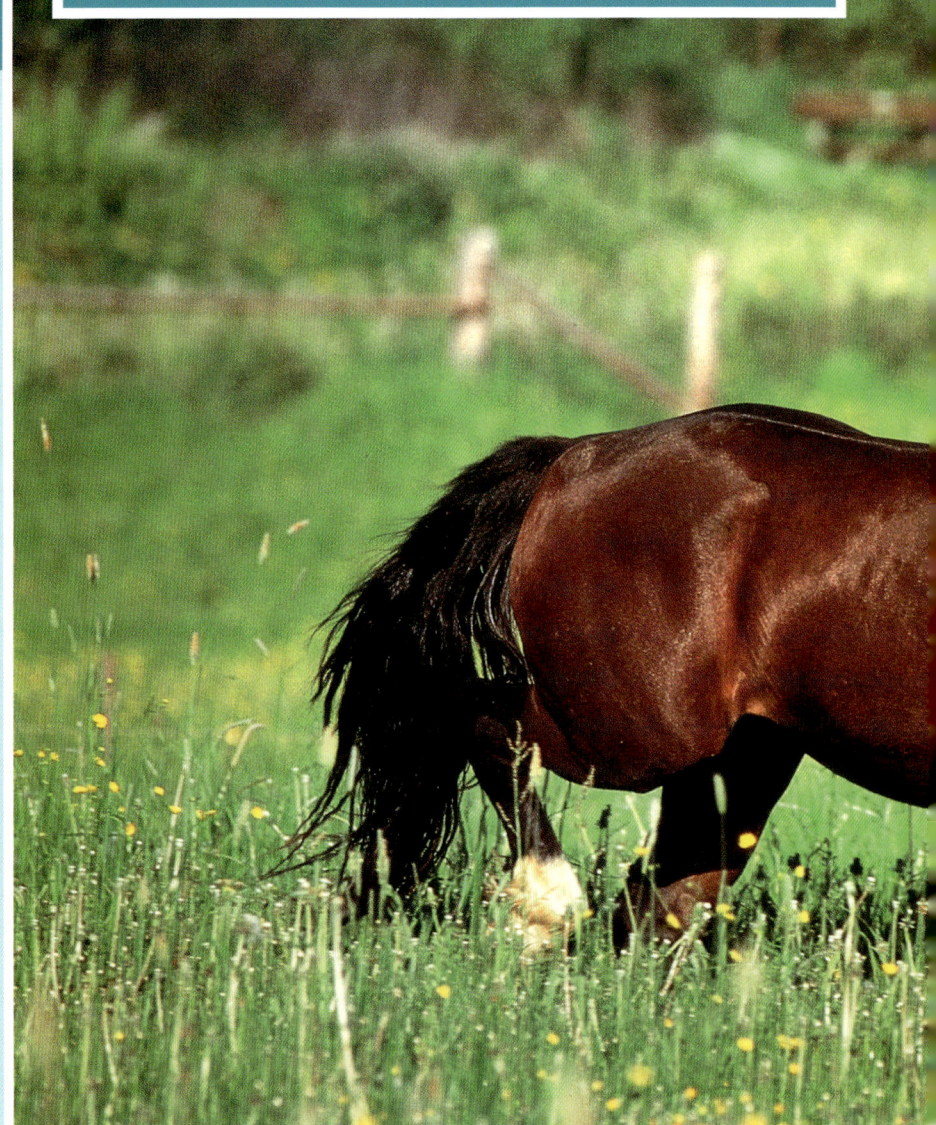

Year-round health

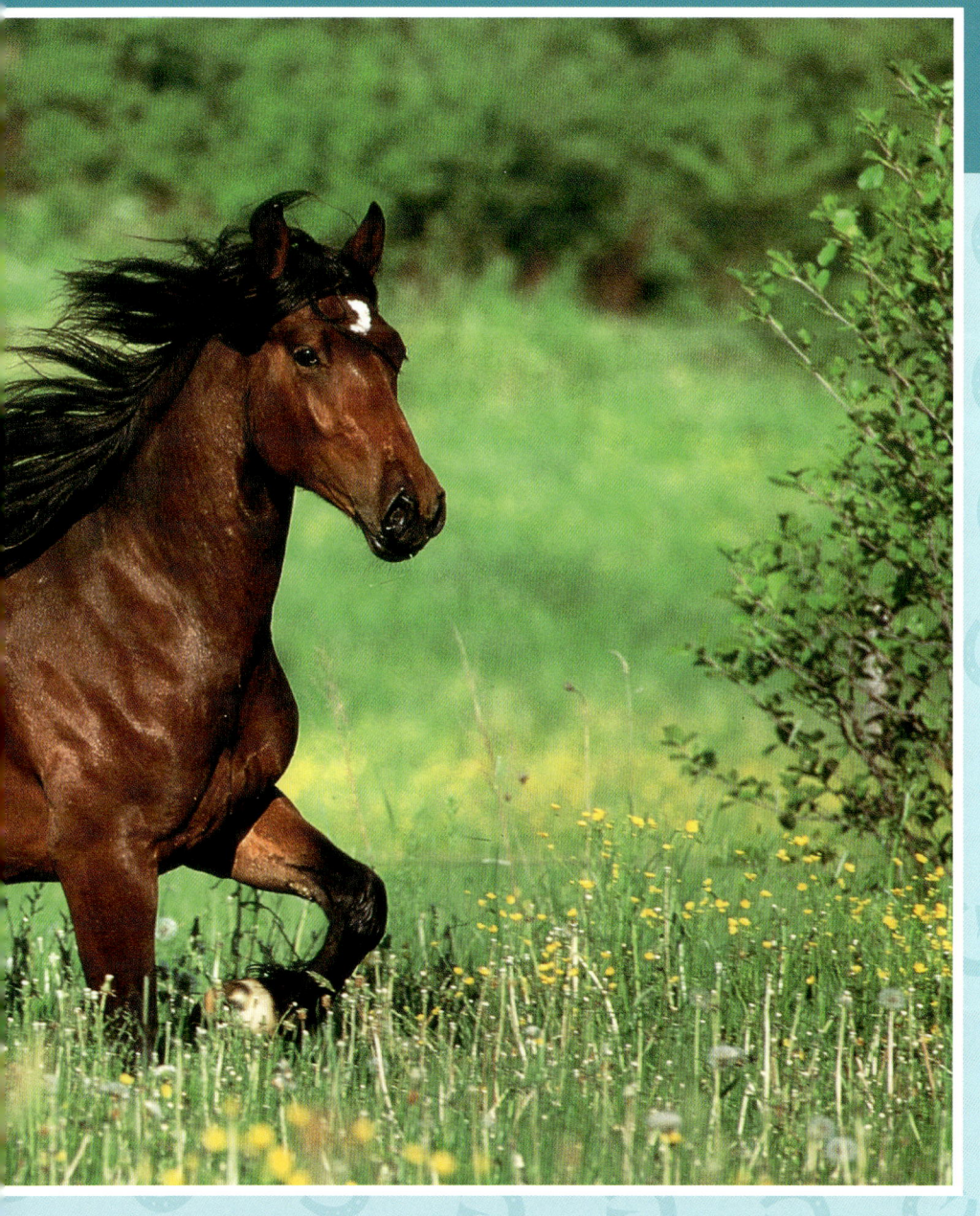

Fresh in the spring

Winter, often very long, is now gone, and nature and our horses are getting ready for spring. The change of coat makes significant demands on the body, often underrated. Horses are more susceptible to infectious diseases, as the lack of sun has weakened the immune system. You should start, no later than February, to facilitate your horses' preparations for spring.

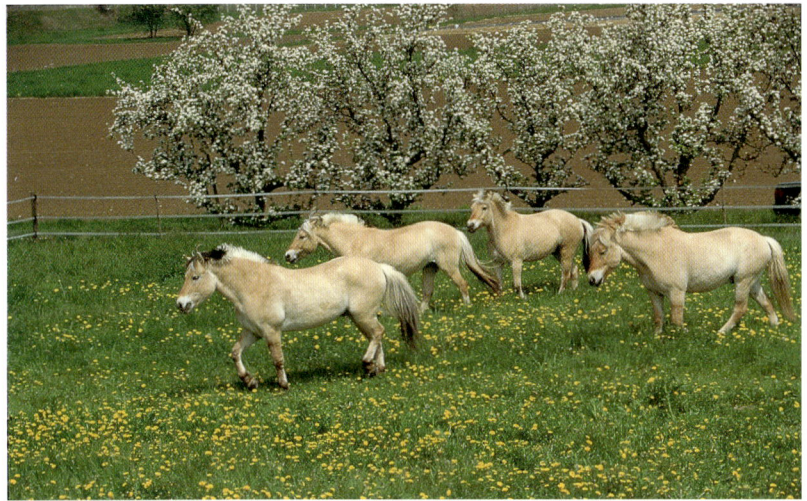

At last cavorting outside again.

Spring fitness course

Horse and rider can undertake a spring fitness course together. Mix a blood-cleansing infusion and pour it over the food once a day. **Nettle, marigold, dandelion, meadowsweet** and **goosegrass**, in addition to cleansing the blood, promote a healthy skin and shiny coat.

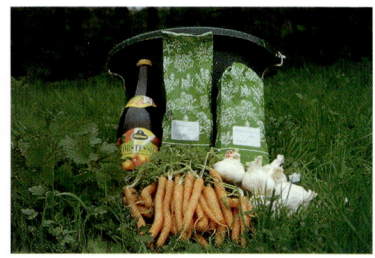

Fit for the spring

If you have not already been giving **garlic** all year round, then it is best to start in the spring. With the first rays of the sun, the midges also begin to dance in the air and the garlic drives them off.

Obviously, **cider vinegar** for horse and rider belongs to any such fitness course. Do you want to be healthy as you ride into the spring? Then every day drink a glass of water with a teaspoon of **honey** and a tablespoon of **vinegar**. Your horse will appreciate this beverage too.

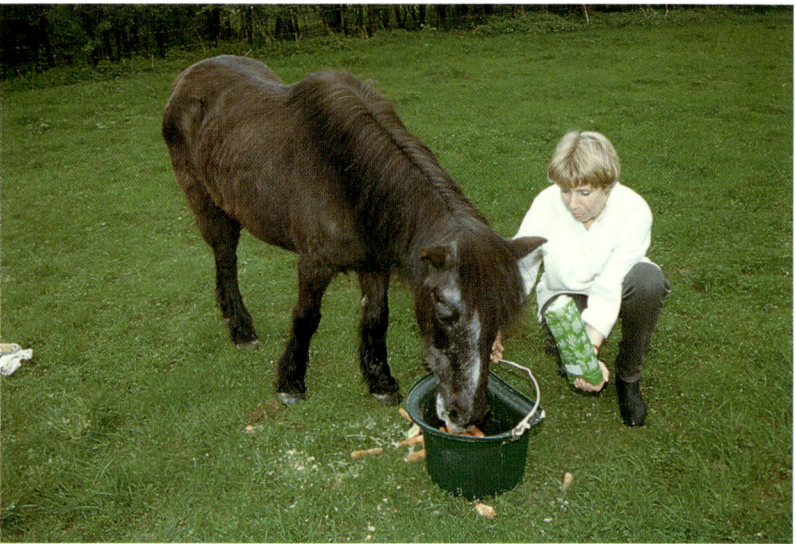

In a spring fitness course, there must be no shortage of carrots, garlic, dandelions . . .

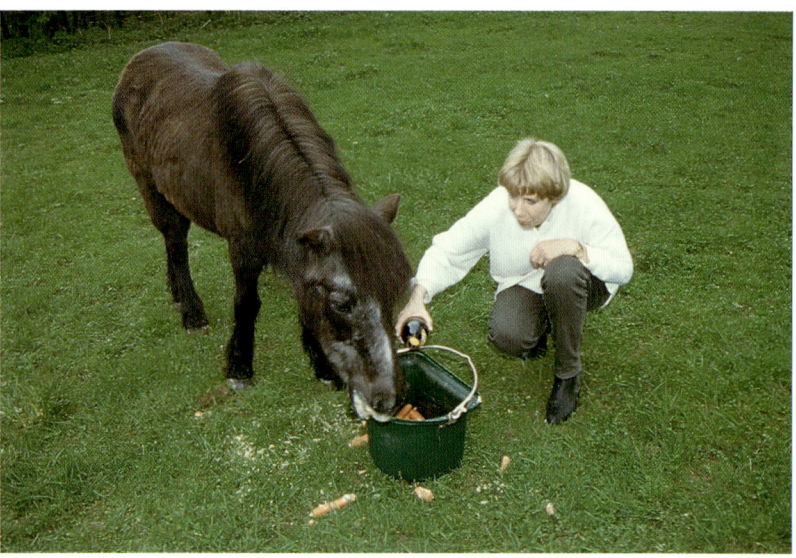

. . . cider vinegar . . .

Grazing time

Horses look forward to the grazing season. But please accustom them slowly to the high-protein spring food. Before being allowed to the pasture, horses should be given concentrated food and hay or straw to ensure that they don't eat the grass too greedily. Mild diarrhoea can be managed with home remedies. **Meadowsweet, anise–fennel–caraway infusion, chamomile, yoghurt** and grated **apples** help to normalise the stools.

Watery diarrhoea, possibly even mixed with blood, is always a case for the vet.

Laminitis

Horses that tend to suffer from laminitis require special attention. My 23-year-old Arabian mare, Kaitra, had very severe laminitis some years ago. In the spring and in September, the pasture is especially rich in protein and I need to be very careful. From February, the mare is given **nettle tea** and twice daily **Ginkgo biloba** for her circulation. These are also beneficial: **garlic, hawthorn leaves, goosegrass** and **comfrey**. I allow Kaitra very early on to graze in a separate section of pasture, when the grass is not yet so lush. During the first few days she is only let out for 20 minutes, then I increase the grazing time slowly.

For horses suffering from laminitis, it is beneficial if you exploit the early morning dew. I used to go for a 30–40 minute walk before 7 a.m. through the tall grass with Kaitra. Movement and cool **water** are beneficial in cases of laminitis.

Keep an eye on your horse. At the slightest sign of awkward movement (stiff gait, 'walking on egg-shells') call a vet or a natural health practitioner. I always keep **Aconitum** and **Nux vomica** in the stable,

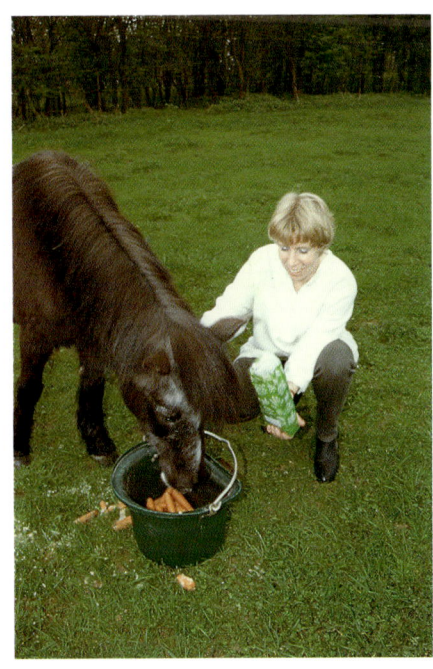

. . . and nettle tea.

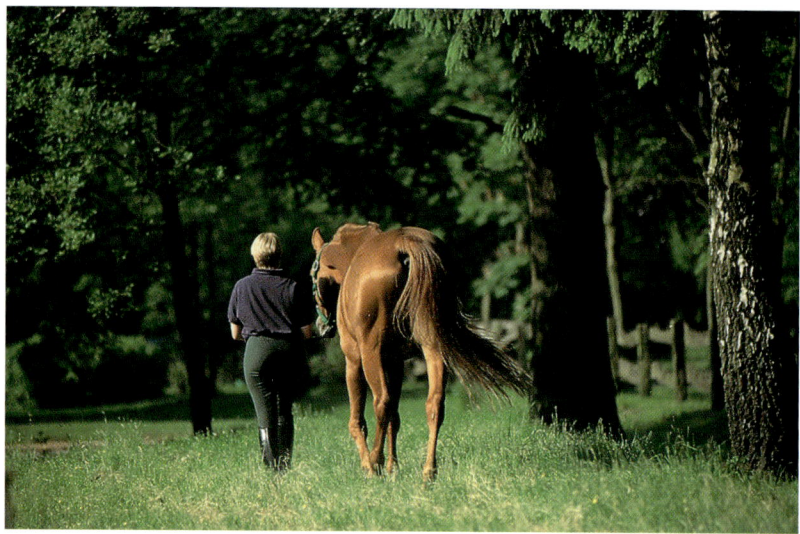

Horses with laminitis need to be in good condition.

two excellent herbal remedies that help the horse alongside the veterinary treatment.

Spring clean

In the case of stabled horses, the change of coat is not as noticeable as in those hardy breeds that spend all of their time outdoors or horses kept in an open barn. Find yourself some time, a place in the sun, a plastic bag for the hairs and a currycomb or exfoliation glove, and help your horse to get rid of the now troublesome winter coat. Our horses enjoy this time of attention and coat care. Make sure that the hairs do not end up in the food or water. A few bunches of hair can be left in hedges, since birds like building their nests with short horse hair. The long hair should be disposed of properly.

As far as possible, try to do the grooming outdoors: the horses see the stable quite enough. Enjoy the spring with a fresh, healthy horse.

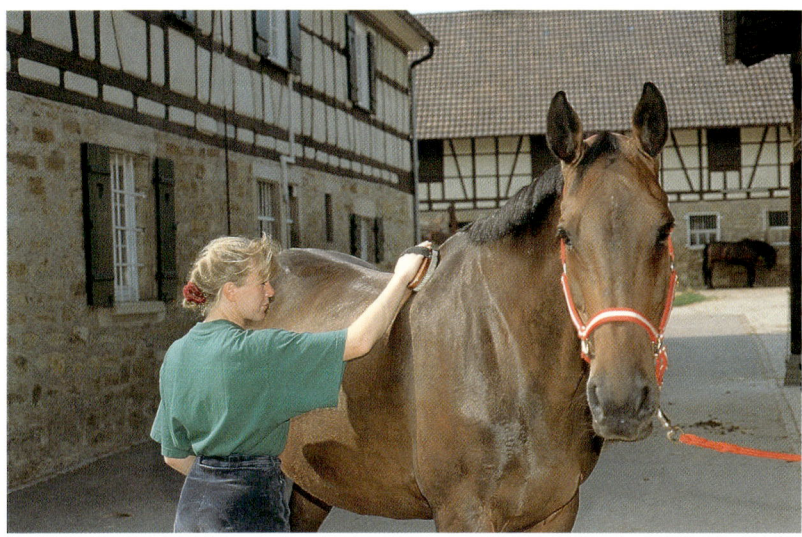

Exfoliation and brushing in the open air are good for the horse's soul, too.

Energy top-up in the summer

Finally the summer is here, and our horses are healthy and beautiful. The coat is shiny, the grazing horses have company, are well-adjusted and content. We look forward to long hacks or to enjoying the tournament season.

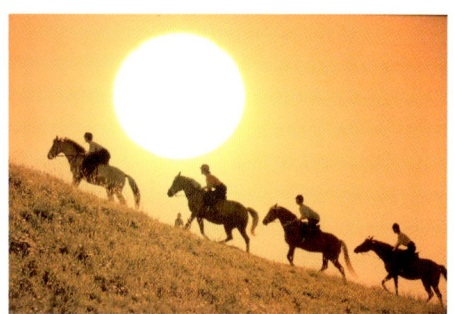

Annoying pests

Unfortunately, the summer has a few downsides too. Above all, this means the flies and midges which make life difficult for horses and also riders. As a preventive, give your horse **cider vinegar** and **garlic**, which put the pests in their place. On very hot days and before a ride, I wash my horses down with **water** and **fruit vinegar**. This treatment keeps them fresh and repels flies. Spraying

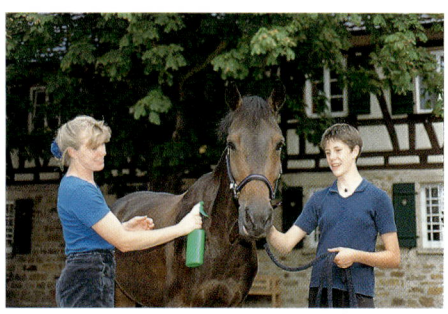

Protection against flies is vital.

with **tea tree** or **eucalyptus oil** is also useful. Hanging a bunch of **lavender** in the stable keeps flies away. **Lavender oil** is also effective when applied to insect bites.

Summer eczema

Horses suffering from eczema need special care. Before sunrise and before sunset they belong in the stable, because of the large number of midges flying about. There are now special protective blankets for summer eczema, and in stubborn cases this is a good solution. Daily washing with **cider vinegar, tea tree oil** or a decoction of **chamomile** and **marigold** can offer help. A **nettle** decoction or infusion is also helpful.

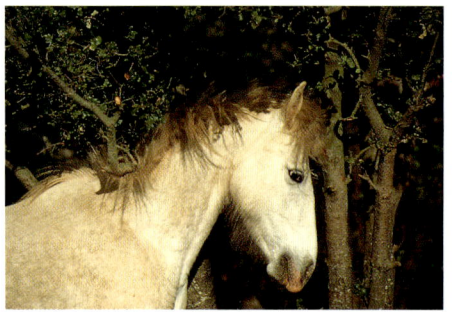

The skin around the mane and tail exhibits areas of scaling and flaking. These respond well to **burdock root oil**. If small areas are scabby or open despite all precautions, they can be treated with oils. The application of **evening primrose oil**, **burdock root oil, avocado oil, apricot oil** and **Aloe vera** will help to remove the scabs and can alleviate itching. Severe cases of summer eczema should always be discussed with the vet.

Any horse suffering from eczema should be well looked after, since it causes itching and chafing.

Cooling off

After a long ride, your horse needs to dry off slowly. Never wash down a hot and sweaty animal with cold water and leave it out in the pasture. Once the horse is dry, brush out the sweat and dust and then wash down the legs and saddle area with **water** and **cider vinegar**, or the whole body if it's a draught-free place. Cool down very tired legs for longer, using a water hose. Do you have a stream in the vicinity? Find a convenient spot and ride through often.

If your horse sweats very quickly and heavily, this may be caused by potassium deficiency which can be helped by eating **bananas**. Especially in the summer, don't forget to provide a salt block so your horse can take up important salts and minerals.

Grazing horses

If your horses gnaw at fences and trees, there are a couple of tried and tested ways to stop this. Rub **lard** into the wood, or even cheaper, coat it with a paste made of **horse droppings** and **water**.

Ponies and horses that spend the whole summer on the pasture should have a daily visit from their rider. We have no wild horses that can manage their life on their own. The hooves have to be inspected briefly every day to check for lodged stones and other foreign objects. When we pass the grooming brush briefly over the horse, we quickly discover small wounds or grazes and can deal with them at an early stage. Warts also occur frequently during the summer. Here, **Thuja** has proved itself an excellent remedy. Thuja as the original mother tincture from the pharmacy, applied externally three to four times a day and 15 drops given internally three times a day, makes almost any wart disappear.

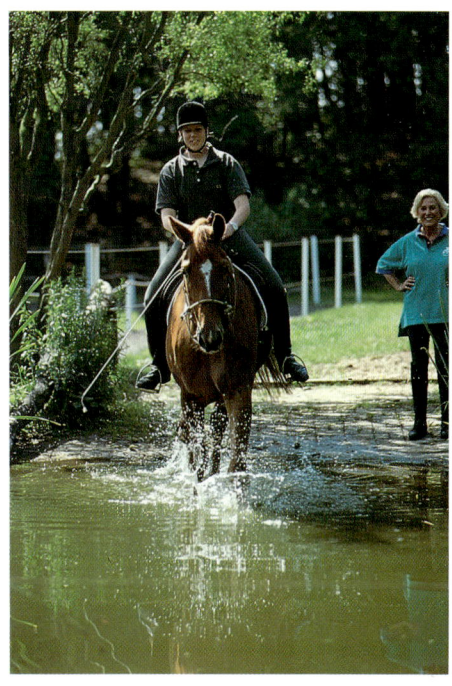

Riding through water is always a welcome refreshment in the summer.

If you are allowed to, collect the droppings as often as you can. This limits worm infestations.

Worming programmes must be carried out regularly throughout the year. Discuss the timetable with your vet. A walk around the meadow will also help discover more quickly any cases of diarrhoea.

Since unfortunately our pastures are no longer herb meadows, naturally herbs can also be added to food during the summer as needed.

All grazing horses should have access to a shelter that is free from flies. Keeping horses unprotected outdoors in the scorching midday sun, at the mercy of flies, borders on cruelty to animals. Sensitive horses can also suffer from sunburn. **Aloe vera** can help here.

Remember that horses too, drink more in hot weather.

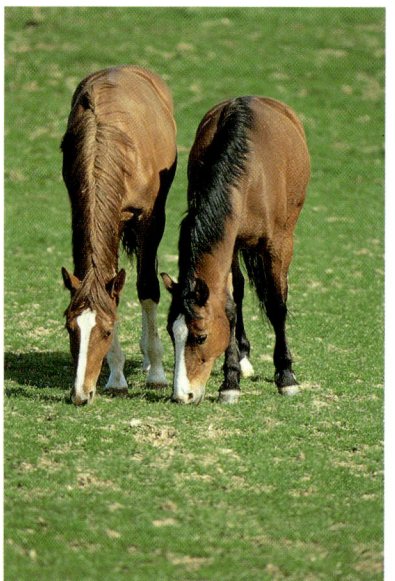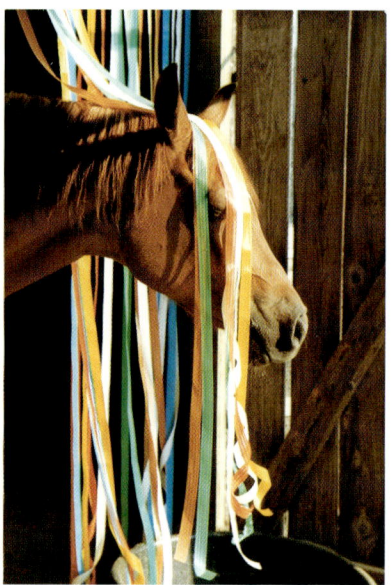

Grazing horses need daily care too . . .   *. . . and a shady shelter free from flies.*

They must always have enough fresh water available, on the pasture and of course also in the stable.

Healthy in the autumn

After a hot summer, often the autumn is the most beautiful time of year. The gentle rays of the sun in a true Indian summer, can offer both horse and rider magical rides. Slowly we get the horses accustomed to different food and to longer stays in the stable.

The change of coat in the autumn is just as taxing for horses as it is in the spring, even if we don't notice it quite as much because of the shorter coat. If the coat is already very thick and the temperatures rise again significantly, often this is quite stressful for the circulation, especially in older horses. In this case, **mistletoe** and **hawthorn** can be very beneficial.

A change of diet

Horses that during the summer were on the pasture day and night and now have to go back to the stable, need to become accustomed slowly to hay and straw. A sudden change of diet can cause constipation colic. To prevent this, look for something in your **tea chest** or add a little **wheat bran**. Bran should always be thoroughly soaked, and you should not feed more than 500 g. Horses that took part in tournaments all summer and still have a few trials ahead

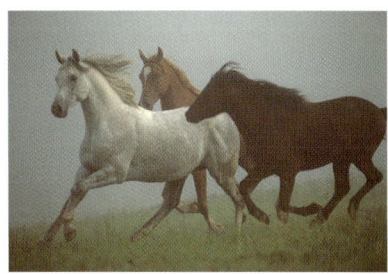

of them, like to have some mash after a strenuous day. You can also prepare ready-bought mash according to the instructions. All horses like mash. If your horse suffers from a lack of appetite due to the change of diet, you can help it with the following recipe: once or twice a week, mix into the mash squashed **juniper berries**, powdered **fenugreek seeds** and **caraway** (one handful in total).

If a horse refuses its food completely, always call a vet at once.

In late summer and autumn, the orchard meadow is a sweet enticement for horses. Within reasonable limits, **pears** and **apples** are a good preparation for the winter. Do, however, check from time to time whether too much is being eaten. Once the horses spend longer periods in the stable, regular feeding with high-moisture food and fruit helps in the changeover from grass to hay and straw.

> **MASH RECIPE**
>
> 1 kg crushed oats
> 800 g bran
> 200 g linseed
> 20 g cooking salt
>
> Pour hot water over the mixture, stir well and let stand until cool enough to be fed by hand.

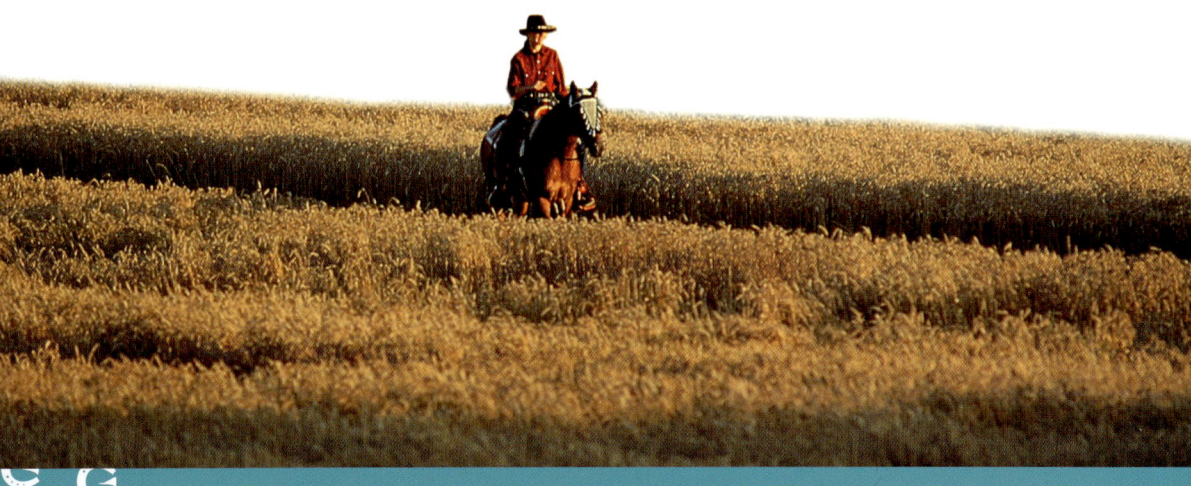

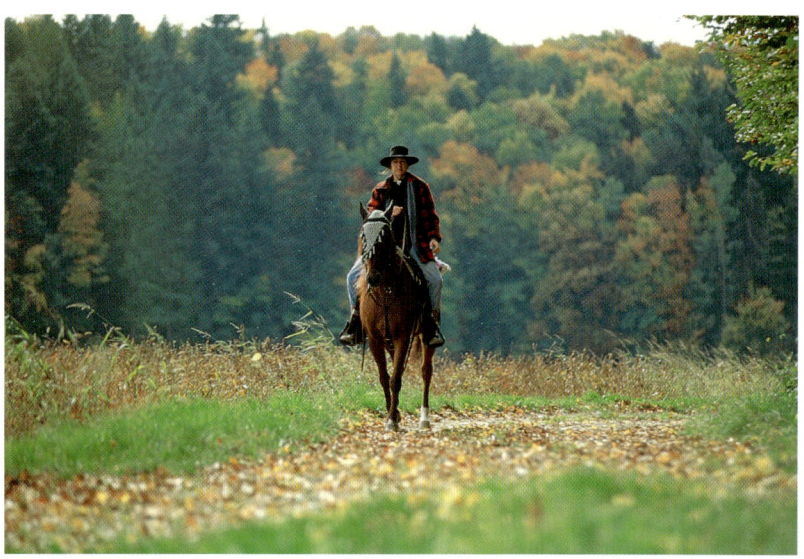

Horse and rider enjoy a hack through the autumnal woods.

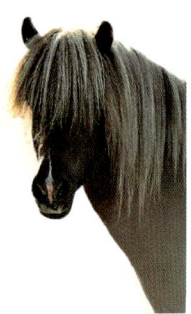

Fit throughout the winter

Horses are physically active animals, not only in the spring, summer and autumn but over their whole lives and throughout the year. Even in winter they need enough open space to run around in, such as a paddock or some other turnout area. All herbal recipes and medicinal remedies will not help if the horses are not kept in proper conditions. A horse needs adequate movement every day.

The right environment

Those who for various reasons cannot keep their horses in an open stable with a paddock for exercise, need to look after them more carefully if they want to have healthy, happy and well-adjusted horses. As soon as you start looking for a stable, you should be thinking about a loose box and a turnout area. The box should be as large as possible. A horse should always be able to observe its peers and the activities in the stable and in the yard. Give your horse **birch branches** and perhaps a ball to play with in the box, since any variety is welcome. When the horses come out of the box, they need to start gradually with a long walk: after all, you too don't embark on a marathon straight after getting out of bed. If there is no possibility of a turnout, the horses should be ridden, lunged or left to run twice a day. If there is a free space or riding hall, let two horses run together: they need the company and should also roll around on the ground.

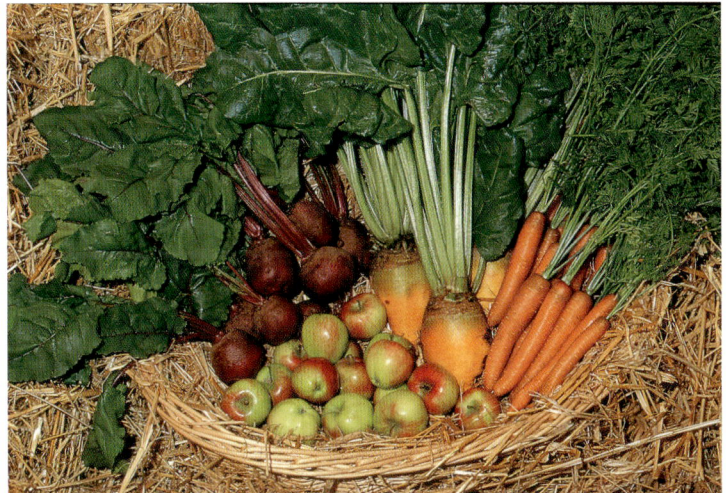

High-moisture food and fruit are especially important in winter.

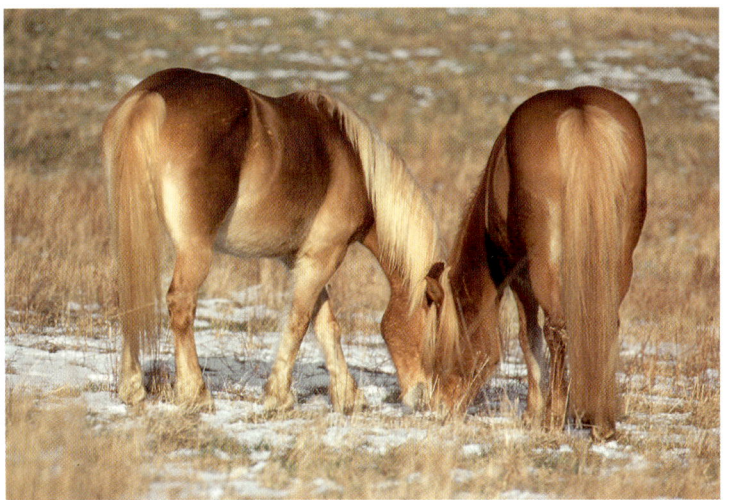

An appropriate turnout should be a matter of course, even in winter.

The right food in winter

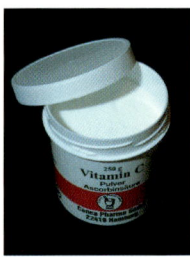

Ascorbic acid is pure vitamin C.

In the box, horses must be provided with enough hay and straw as rough-age, and with concentrated food at least three times a day. High-moisture food and fruit offer additional variety and regulate the digestion.

Teatime is especially indicated during the cold time of year. In winter, my horses are given a **tea** to drink at least once a day. Fortify the horses' immune system with **cider vinegar** and perhaps **ascorbic acid** (vitamin C). In powder form, one teaspoon is enough.

More than anything else, coughs bother horses a lot in winter. Mix together some herbs and give the horses an inhalation. A **cough infusion** has also proven effective in my horses.

Elderly horses

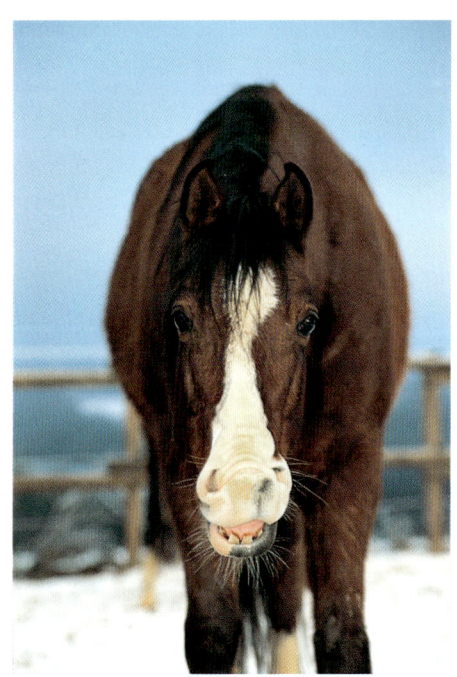

Elderly horses benefit in winter from a hot meal with various herbs.

Older horses especially, need more care and attention in winter. For many years they have made our lives better, and now are entitled to make greater demands on our time. Often they can no longer get the full value out of food, and their metabolism too doesn't work too well. I am always happy when I get my older horses through the winter again. Our Polly is going on for 40, and my Arabian mare is 23.

When it's really cold, the older horses get a **mash meal** twice a week, and various **infusions** over the food as needed. When it's frosty, I warm up the drinking water in the morning and check a couple of times a day whether it has frozen. **Garlic** and **cider vinegar** are given all year round. You can enrich the winter diet with dried **nettles**. Horses can also tolerate well one egg per day. Feed the egg with the shell crushed finely, the calcium is good for the hooves and coat. **Beetroot** is an additional source of vitamins. One or two pots of **yoghurt** are read-ily eaten if given with **honey** or mixed into the mash.

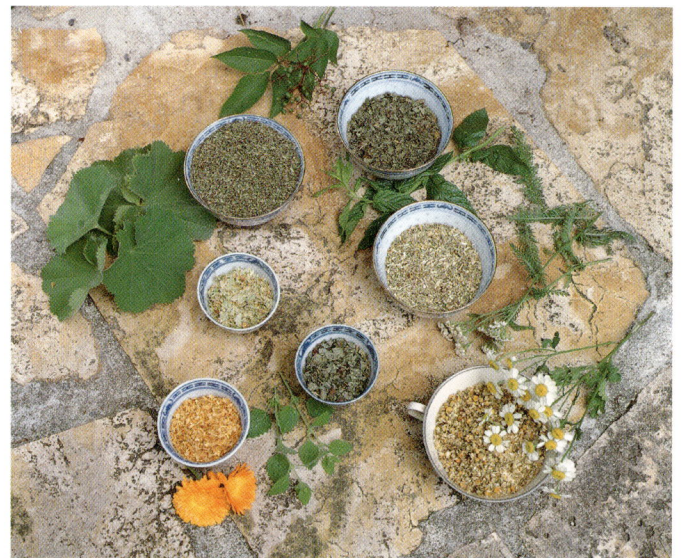

Chamomile, yarrow, marigold and so on are especially important in winter.

Malanders in winter

Since our leisure horses have open stabling with a turnout all year round, I need not worry about exercise and contact with other horses. When it snows, sometimes I can't tear myself away, it's too much fun to watch how the sprightly old-age pensioners, spurred on by the cold-blood Alma, cavort through the snow and become young again.

However, in winter one often struggles with malanders, especially in horses kept in open stabling. Good hoof care and dry legs are important. In addition to veterinary treatment, one can give **Thuja** (mother tincture) twice or three times a day, drizzled on a piece of bread.

Massage **burdock root oil** on the clean, dry skin. The hooves can be rubbed with pure **laurel oil**. Massage the oil carefully with a toothbrush into the coronet. If you try a few of these tips, you will surely keep your horses in top condition through the winter.

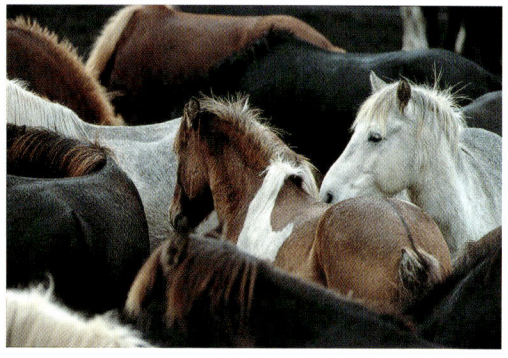

In winter too, horses can be outdoors during the day.

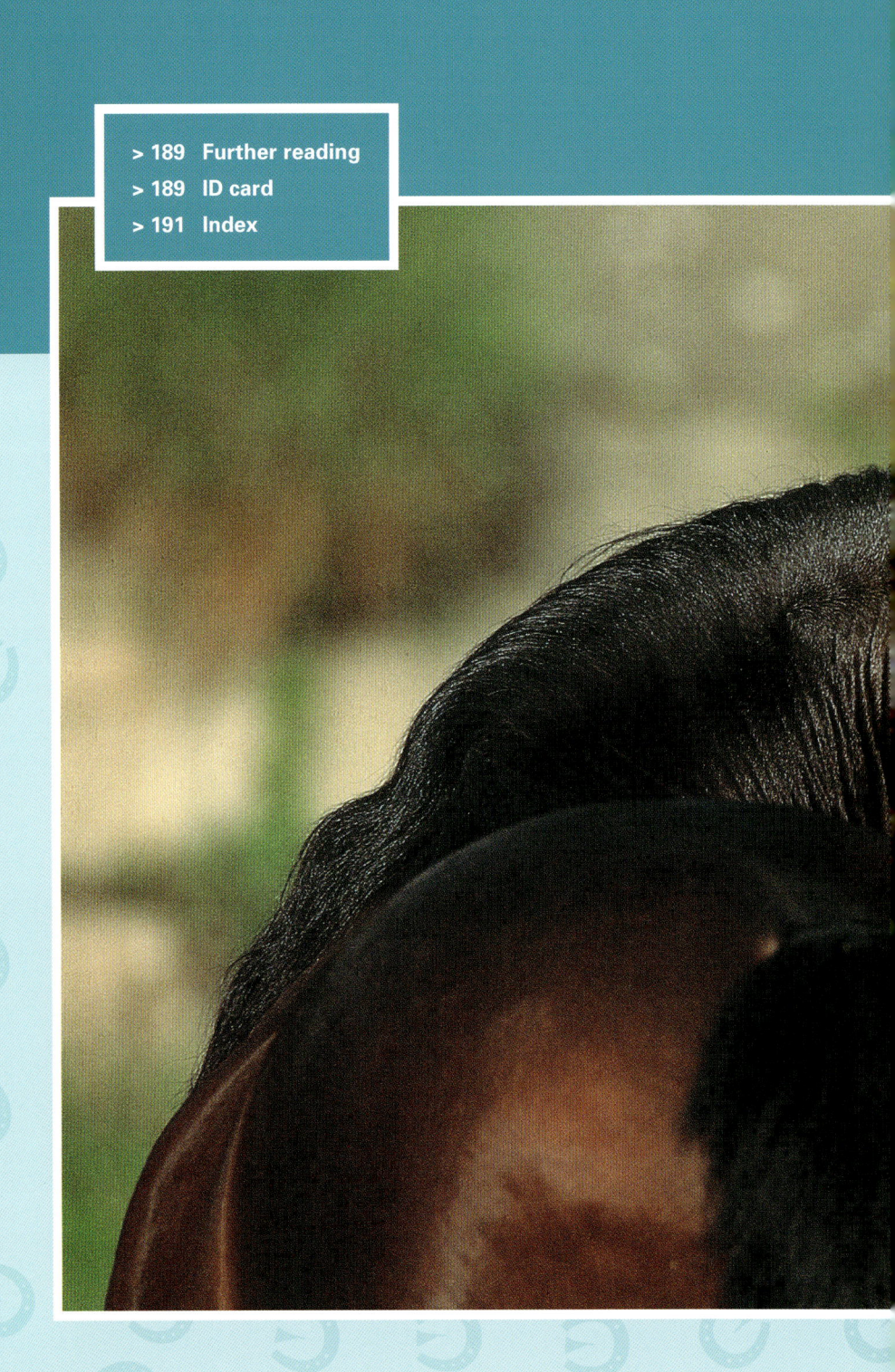

Miscellaneous

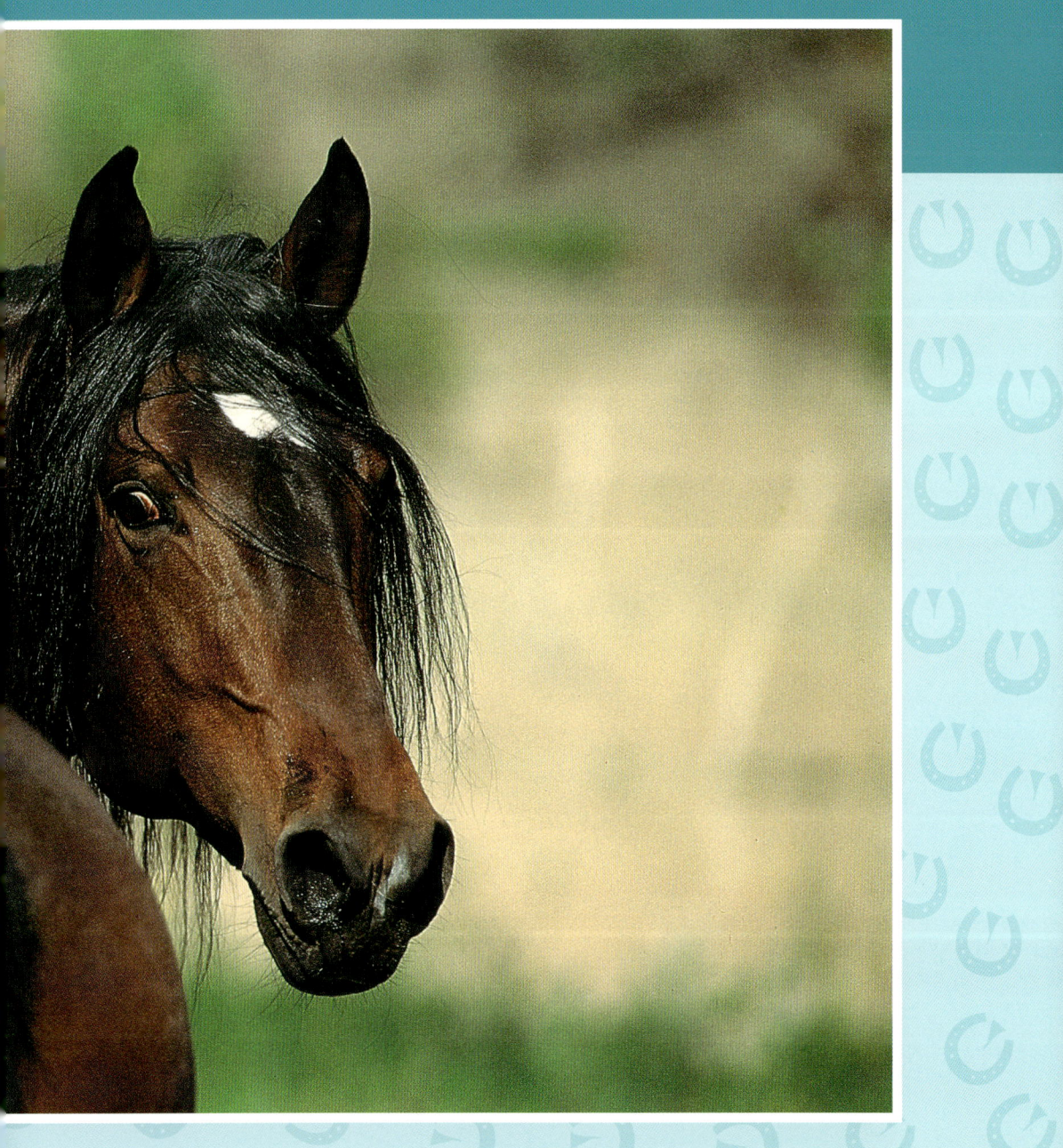

Further reading – Horse riding and management series

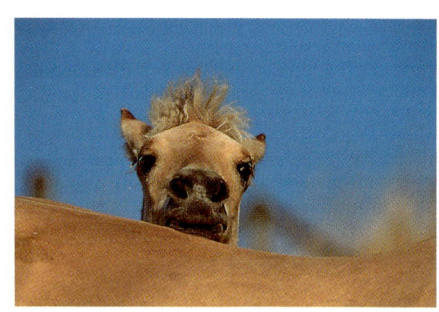

Foals and Young Horses: Training and Management for a Well-Behaved Horse by Ute Ochsenbauer and Beate Schmidtlein

Horse Behaviour: Interpreting the Horse's Body Language and Communication by Barbara Schöning

ID card

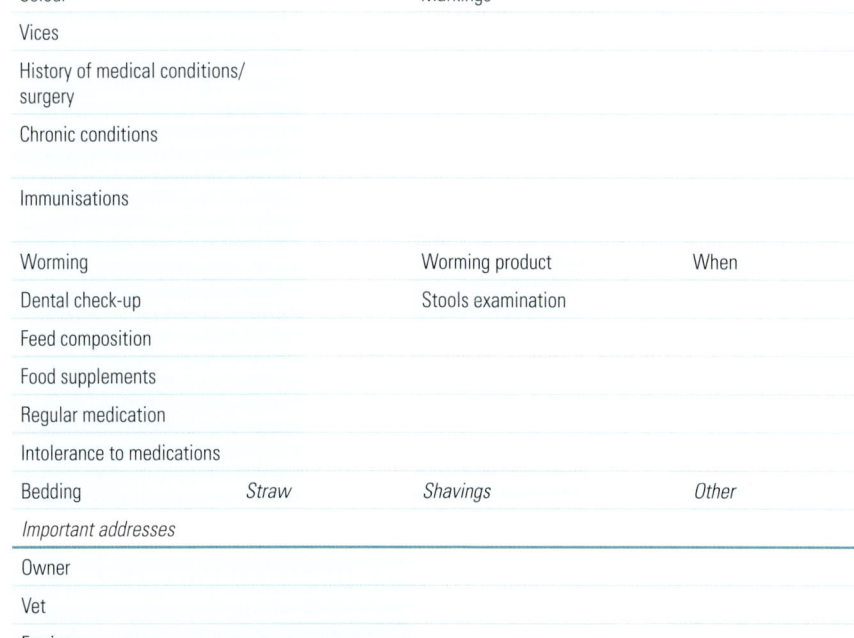

Name		
Date of birth	Sex	
Leisure horse	Competition Horse	
Breed	Height	
Colour	Markings	
Vices		
History of medical conditions/ surgery		
Chronic conditions		
Immunisations		
Worming	Worming product	When
Dental check-up	Stools examination	
Feed composition		
Food supplements		
Regular medication		
Intolerance to medications		
Bedding	*Straw*	*Shavings*	*Other*
Important addresses		
Owner		
Vet		
Farrier		
Stable		
Emergency services		

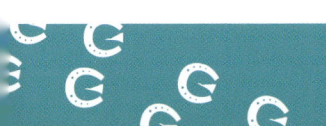

Index

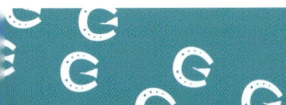